Praise for *Baby Om*

"A splendidly well-written guide of yoga postures for new mums and their infants. The thoughtfulness, knowledge, and caring come through on each page. A wonderful book."

—Carol Foster, prenatal yoga teacher

"A lovely gift to mothers and babies everywhere. Combining their extensive and rigorous yoga backgrounds with their warm and accessible style, the authors have created a unique and meaningful way for mothers to connect with their babies and to reconnect with themselves in body, mind, and spirit."

—Aly Mandel, Baby Om student and clinical psychologist

"This book addresses with great insight how to incorporate a new baby into one's yoga practice."

—Genevieve Kapuler, certified Iyengar yoga teacher

"Baby Om is the single best thing I have done for my babies and myself in the past two and a half years. Laura and Sarah's practical approach and down-to-earth advice helped turn this exhausted and out-of-shape mum into one with more energy and a greater appreciation of my body. Even better, I was able to share this amazing experience with my children."

—Alyssa Gilbert, Baby Om student and cognitive therapist

"The first time I opened the book I could not stop smiling. It is creative, inventive, intelligent, and most of all fun! I will share it with all my students—men and women of all ages, just for the inspiration of new life."

—Jeanne-Marie Derrick, Iyengar yoga instructor

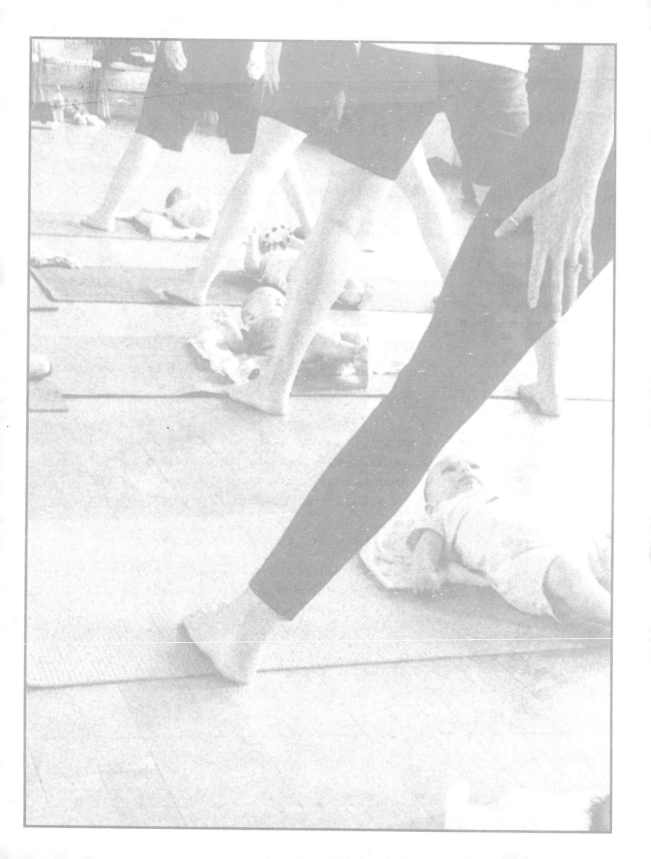

Baby Om

Yoga for Mothers and Babies

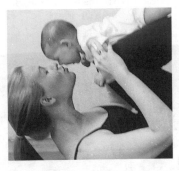

LAURA STATON *and* SARAH PERRON

Newleaf

Published in Ireland by
Newleaf
an imprint of
Gill & Macmillan Ltd
Hume Avenue, Park West, Dublin 12
with associated companies throughout the world
www.gillmacmillan.ie
Copyright © 2002, 2003 by Laura Staton and Sarah Perron
0 7171 3565 9
First published in the United States of America 2002 by
Henry Holt and Company, LLC, New York
Printed by ColourBooks Ltd, Dublin

The paper used in this book comes from the wood pulp of managed forests.
For every tree felled, at least one tree is planted, thereby renewing natural resources.

A CIP catalogue record for this book is available from the
British Library.

1   3   5   4   2

To

Rosey and Dylan

with love

You started it all.

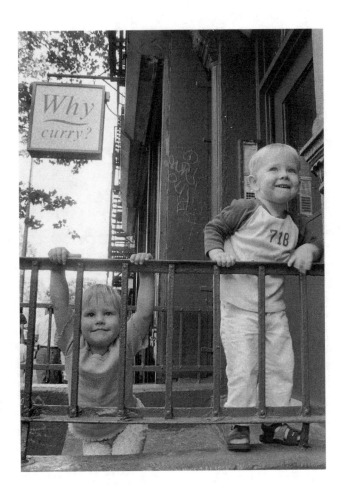

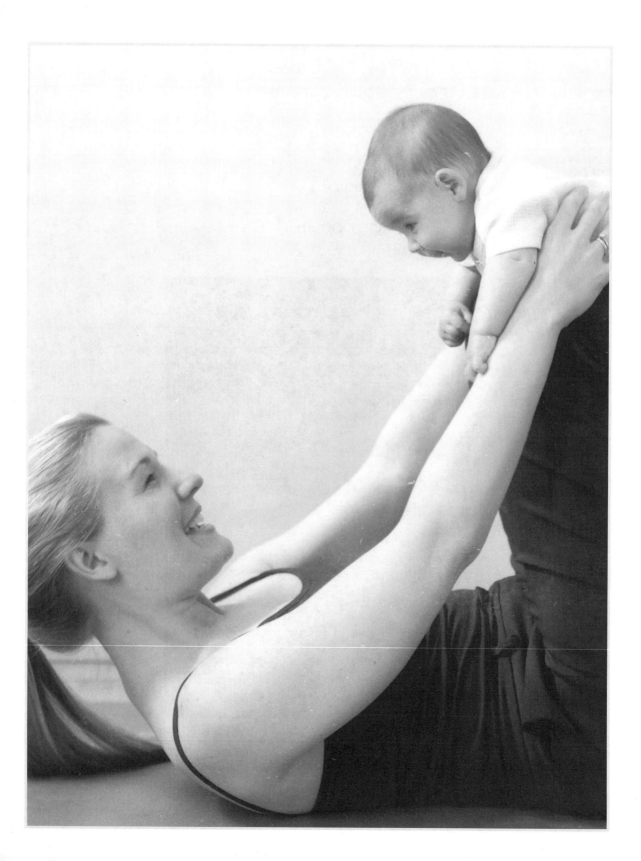

Contents

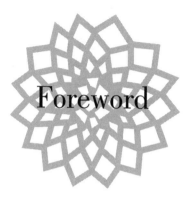

Foreword

In the first few days, weeks, and months of an infant's life, mother and baby learn to adjust to each other in creating their relationship. It is a kind of yoga: the one has become two, and the two spontaneously create a union that establishes something greater than there was before. Within this primary matrix, the foundation is set for the infant's growing individuality to emerge—"This is my hand touching your face"—and the experience of becoming a separate self is set in motion. From these ongoing interactions, the mother-child relationship grows.

It is at this pivotal time in development that a mother must be present and receptive to the needs of her baby. It is, however, often a time when she may feel exhausted and stressed. This is reflected at every level of experience. Physically, her body can lack agility and seem as though it is not her own. How, then, can a mother feel receptive to the needs of her baby when she may not be in harmony with herself? How can she nurture another when she feels so overwhelmed?

With their deep understanding of the conditions essential for healthy union, Sarah Perron and Laura Staton have created a sequence of carefully designed yoga poses that heighten a woman's awareness of her body and allow her to gently open and come into the present. With these subtle yet profound changes of her body, Mum begins to experience a developing confidence. As she nurtures herself, she becomes more in touch with her own needs, enabling her to be more sensitive to the needs of her infant. Because the baby is an eager participant in every Baby Om class, the possibilities of connection between the two are heightened in unique ways.

Although mothers gain greater resilience and vitality as they progress, the class is not just for them. And, though the babies appear to be having a wonderful time, the class is not just for them, either. Instead, each class is geared toward enhancing the developing relationship. Whether the baby is hoisted on Mum's hip as a part of her Warrior pose, placed belly down on the mat as a reflection of her Cobra pose, or guided through a series of baby poses, the potential for each partner to gracefully merge with, then separate from the other is enhanced. Through a variety of these yogic activities, the mother-baby relationship grows in flexibility and receptivity—the roots of good health.

Besides all that, it's fun!

RUELLA FRANK, PH.D.
PSYCHOLOGIST, INFANT EDUCATOR,
AND YOGA PRACTITIONER

INTRODUCTION:

The Baby Om Story

When people ask us why we created a business of mother and baby yoga classes two months into parenthood, we have to be honest: we did it because we needed them. As new mothers we hardly felt like budding entrepreneurs. We were elated and exhausted, and most of all felt an overwhelming urge to spend time with our children. But as women, as dancers, and as yoga teachers, we yearned to get back into shape. Learning how to practice yoga along with our babies turned out to be the only way to indulge both needs: to deepen our bonds with our children while healing our postpartum selves physically and mentally. And by creating classes for others around what we learned—classes that turned into *Baby Om*—we managed to help a network of mothers and friends do the same. We wrote this book hoping it will do the same for you.

Why does yoga, more than any other form of exercise, address the needs of new mothers so well? We'll explore this question in more detail later on, but there's a simple answer. Yoga is all about flexibility—in addressing your changing life as well as your stiff limbs! It stretches and strengthens you, gently assisting a gradual return to physical strength just as it can deliver a shattering

1

workout. It encourages improvisation and play. It provides babies with a soothing environment in which to begin experiencing their bodies' interactions with the world. So it perfectly answers the new mother's need for a calming yet rigorous way to align and strengthen her body while still having fun with her baby. Throughout our pregnancies we suspected some of this. After all, we were yoga teachers and felt that yoga would be an integral part of our early parenthood. We just had no idea how much it would help, or that a new business and a new life for both of us would result.

Our friendship is based on our shared passions. We followed parallel career paths that started in modern dance and embraced teaching yoga as a (slightly) less impoverishing profession. When we each found out we were pregnant, we were elated, but also uncertain about the future. How would we combine the physical demands of our professional lives with the needs of our children so that no one felt shortchanged? Sarah, who had toured with Mikhail Baryshnikov, was pregnant with Rosey and was still dancing and directing rehearsals for the company she had performed with for over a decade. Laura, who had been choreographing and dancing since leaving Juilliard, was pregnant with Dylan and had a full calendar of dance commitments. Still worse, we were both scheduled to perform in a show around two months after our babies were due. What were we thinking?

While we danced and taught through our ninth month, our birth experiences turned out to be very different. Laura underwent a difficult labor that ended with a cesarean section, while Sarah had an unmedicated vaginal delivery. Both of us emerged as delighted and depleted as every new mother. But after a two-month blur of diaper changes, family visits, midnight feedings, and baby vomit, the dreaded show arrived. While our husbands in the audience nervously held fussing babies, we staggered and finessed our way through the whole thing. Backstage between dances and impromptu feedings, we tried to calm our anxiety and catch our breath, but the reality was obvious: life had changed, and so had we. It was time to get back in shape.

The next week we began searching the city for yoga classes we could take with our babies in tow. What we found wasn't promising. Our first instinct was to return to our usual yoga classes, an everyday routine before we had babies. But since those classes are far from baby-friendly, we were faced with either leaving our newborns with a friend or family member (a favor quickly used up) or finding a baby-sitter (costly). There were also postpartum classes that included babies but these tended either to concentrate mainly on the infant (baby massage, for example) or offered meditative yoga focusing on breathing and soothing. While we wanted to include our babies, we still craved a complete workout—one tailored to our postpartum bodies, aimed at strengthening, aligning, and grounding. The combination simply wasn't to be found.

One day, sitting around Laura's apartment eating jellybeans, it dawned on us that since we couldn't find the class we wanted, we should create one. We could construct exactly the environment that we knew we, as new mums, wanted and that others might want, too: a class that would address mothers and babies equally, a class applicable to anyone, from swami to couch potato. We decided to give it a go. We rented studio space, took our kids and yoga mats along, and began to experiment several times a week with what felt right for our bodies, our psyches, and our infants.

The joy of discovering a robust physical activity that we could share with a tiny, fragile infant was tremendous. We found focus and energy. We uncovered an entirely new way of playing with Rosey and Dylan: we could fly them on our knees while strengthening our abdominal muscles; we could breathe through warm-ups like Sun Salutes while tickling them; we could exercise their tiny limbs and enjoy their smiling response. Our mother-child bonds deepened. The babies also got to know each other, becoming close friends who shared everything from pacifiers to partially chewed bagels. Each time we left the studio, regardless of the amount of yoga we actually got to practice, we felt better about ourselves. These sessions became the highlight of the spring and summer of 1999.

That September, with some trepidation, we launched Baby Om with a class that was attended by one mother, Naomi. Since then, the response of our students has been tremendous. To our surprise, we've started amassing the trappings of a "real" business, including a great logo designed by our friend Victoria Lewis, and the now-obligatory Web site (www.babyom.com). We have also experimented with two variations on the original Baby Om concept: Toddler Om (a riotous failure) and prenatal classes (a great success). We are most proud, however, of the individual success stories of which we are privileged to have been part.

One of our current students, Andrea, is a great example. She had a difficult birth and found that yoga was the only exercise she and her baby, Katie, were able to do. *"Katie loved it from day one. She became relaxed, and then I was able to focus on what I needed to do."* She now practices daily, finding that yoga helps build her confidence and patience.

Susan, a Web designer who works from home, was thrilled to be able to spend time concentrating on her second child, Trygve, as she worked out. She was also excited to learn that we had designed a yoga class to do while nursing.

Judy recalls being afraid to move herself or her child until she started Baby Om and how the classes helped her become more physically secure both in her own body and when handling her daughter.

Best of all, most students can't believe how great they feel after each class. Whether they were in great shape before the baby arrived or not, yoga helps them find a sense of their former selves. Postpartum mothers will be flushed with excitement from suddenly finding themselves touching their toes for the first time since their second trimester. They are always far more surprised than we are. Other parents, distraught over their apparently inconsolable crying kids, are thrilled weeks later when their babies have calmed and are gurgling and shrieking with delight. Once they are used to the classes, babies will roll, crawl, start fledgling conversations, engage in small battles over toys, or burble along while the adults chant.

Some parents tell us how much their babies look forward all week to coming to class. We often wonder how the babies communicate this. In any event, whether they actually looked forward to class or not, we have graduated hundreds of babies since our opening. As for their caregivers, though our students are most often first-time mothers, we have taught all kinds of people: fathers, gay and lesbian couples, and even grandparents. One new mother regularly brought her own mother to class, which gave us the pleasure of watching three generations practice yoga together, each mum relating to her daughter from a different perspective. We find that non-birth parents often value the interactive time spent with the baby more than the yoga itself; they find that yoga contributes a language of physical bonding to their relationship. Classes also provide students a chance to meet a network of other parents and share experiences in a small, intimate setting that embraces their children. The value of this network is enhanced by the variety of our students' professions: doctors, photo editors, analysts, writers, social workers, designers, office managers, lawyers, and models, to name only a few. We've even taught some fellow dancers!

We never expected any of this to happen; we were just looking for a class to fill our needs. Somewhere along the way we were lucky enough to join a growing and loving community of parents and babies who come together to share the joy and restorative power of yoga.

How to Use This Book

What *Baby Om* offers is a comprehensive method for achieving flexibility and strength and deepening your knowledge of your body and baby. Don't think, however, that this will somehow be second best compared to actually taking one of our classes. While we're great advocates of classes, it's also important to stress that one of the fundamental goals of yoga is to develop a personal practice. Perhaps as important, doing yoga at home has many practical advantages if you have a new baby. You can go at your own pace, paying attention to your specific areas of need. You can choose the ideal moment for your class—always helpful when negotiating unpredictable nap times! You don't have to waste precious time on travel. And you don't have to go it alone—you can practice with friends or even create your own group.

We've organized the book around you and your child's development. First, we address some necessary fundamentals: chapter 1, "What's So Great about Yoga?," explores the benefits of yoga; chapter 2, "Baby Om Basics," lays out all the practical information you need to get going; and chapter 3, "Baby Engagement," deals with playing and stimulating your baby during yoga. After that comes the core of the book: four yoga classes, each concentrating on a unique stage in your child's growth and your recovery during the first year after birth.

Class 1: This class for the first three months of your baby's life is for everyone from beginner on. It addresses basic postpartum needs such as restoring core alignment and beginning to strengthen and reconnect overstretched pelvic floor and abdominal muscles. It's designed to nourish your body and mind with much-needed calm. The baby exercises will gently stimulate your infant's body, basic motor skills, and vision.

Class 2: This class covers months three to six and is aimed at a slightly more intermediate level. It focuses on some wonderful chest-opening positions that will lift your spirits and stretch those tight shoulders. By this time you'll be getting stronger, and you'll become able to exert yourself without as much potential for exhaustion. Your baby will be stronger, perhaps attempting the Cobra pose (tummy down, head lifted), and will probably sit with assistance.

Class 3: Addressing months six to twelve, this class enables you to engage in a more vigorous practice. By this time you'll be physically stronger and well on your way to a more balanced and integrated body, so this class is more varied and strenuous than the first two. Your baby will now be using you as a personal jungle gym, excitedly practicing pulling, crawling, and assisted walking. This class will get you and keep you in good enough shape to run after and carry your baby without strain.

Class 4: This class addresses the unique needs of mothers who underwent a cesarean section, and runs in parallel chronologically with Class 1 (0–3 months). It is designed to accommodate a high level of physical tenderness and even discomfort, focusing on gently strengthening the post-surgery body. It is also recommended to any mother as a restorative class to take when feeling especially frayed around the edges. The infant exercises described in Class 1 apply here, albeit with some added caution to avoid straining the incision site. Please note that if you had a C-section we recommend you start this class no sooner than six weeks after giving birth.

The four class chapters are followed by discussions of different aspects of yoga and motherhood, including yoga for nursing and to soothe colic, yoga and postpartum depression, and the process and physical effects of childbirth.

The later chapters include a certain amount of medical information, some of it technical—and we think it's important they do. In our experience, it really helps your yoga practice if you understand the dramatic physical impact of pregnancy and birth. We have tried to do this in a medical context that addresses specific health issues with clarity. Just use the information that interests you or is pertinent to your body.

In terms of when it's safe to start *asana* practice (that is, active exercise), if you've had a vaginal birth we recommend that you wait three or four weeks after delivery (assuming all bleeding has stopped), and if you've had a cesarean section we recommend that you wait six weeks and that you get your doctor's approval before starting. Each class has a suggested breathing practice that you can start earlier, beginning around ten days after birth. Kegel exercises can be done as soon as three days after a vaginal birth. Working the pelvic floor muscles brings fresh oxygenated blood to the tissues to promote healing, especially if you've had tearing or an episiotomy. We also recommend that you take things slowly: work on Class 1 or the cesarean Class 4 for the full three months before moving ahead to the other chapters, even if you feel you've mastered the poses. After the changes and challenges producing a baby, your body deserves a gentle and balanced recovery period.

The baby exercises suggested in each chapter should be introduced during that particular period in your child's development. It's best not to rush ahead, since they are designed to address specific developmental phases. You can accumulate a repertoire of exercises and mix familiar elements in with the new, but we don't recommend challenging your three-month-old with the exercises for a nine-month-old!

What yoga can provide for you is a practice that will help you develop a sensitivity toward your body. Let this sensitivity inform your practice as you learn to trust your physical instincts.

Think of the classes as recipes for you and your baby. We hope you take what is useful, are inspired by what may seem unfamiliar, and, most important, fit a little yoga into your life.

Welcome to *Baby Om*.

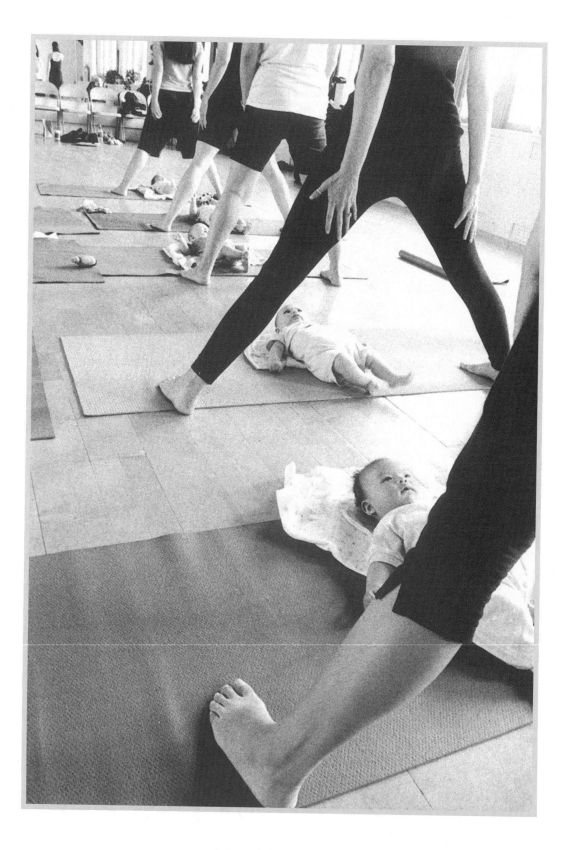

1
What's So Great about Yoga?

Yoga with babies? To some people yoga might seem like a completely natural thing to do with your infant. To others it makes as much sense as teaching her the jitterbug. Yoga teachers often talk about overcoming your own self-imposed limits. As parents we often try to do the same thing. Yoga encourages us to look beyond our assumed boundaries, both physical and emotional. Limitations—self-imposed or dictated by external conditions—are all around us, and it's hard not to cling to ideas, especially when it comes to raising children. Often we have more choices than we think.

Yoga practice encourages you to go deeper into your physical self where you may bump up against your own assumptions about your limitations only to find they are ideas, not necessarily hard facts. Flexibility, a core tenet of yoga practice, means giving new ideas a chance to prove themselves or being open to alternative ways to instill the kinds of habits you want for your child and for yourself.

What do we think about when we think about yoga? Most people will say it has something to do with connecting the mind and body, and as dancers we were drawn to yoga in part because of this simple definition. We found that yoga practice had a lot in common with dance. Both involve physicality and precision, strengthening your limbs and stretching the spine, and exploring space and the individual experience of time. It was never boring.

But what is yoga, exactly? You probably know the basics: it's a 5,000-year-old spiritual practice begun in India, based on the knowledge that the physical, emotional, and spiritual elements of life are inseparable and ever-changing. There are many aspects of yoga, one of which is *asana* practice. *Asanas* are physical movements or poses that can be combined in different ways to provide a range of benefits. Through these poses, yoga encourages an inquiring approach to the body, meeting a variety of musculoskeletal, meditative, organic, and energetic needs. *Asana* asks that you go inward, learn to concentrate on the connection between breathing, your physical self, your thoughts and feelings.

Most important, yoga also meets you at your level, which is why it's the ideal postpartum exercise. You can begin yoga at any time in your life and it is a diverse enough practice to encompass an enormous range of physical experience. Yoga can be gentle, but it is also a form of rigorous exercise, and it's worth noting that yoga was originally done exclusively by young men. Only in the twentieth century did renowned yoga schools in India begin to admit women. Today the practice has spread around the world and yoga practitioners come in all shapes, sizes, genders, and ages—even babies.

Baby Om was designed to be a serious yoga class for the postpartum body that includes the baby as well. What happens in a baby yoga class? Interaction. Communication. Touch, play, and fun. You are encouraged to get down on the floor and interact with your baby as an equal. The physical aspect of yoga can calm you so you are more available to yourself and your child. You experience the present moment—something your baby does automatically. This is a wonderful way to get to know your child. That's why we do yoga with our babies instead of lifting weights, riding a stationary bike, or jogging.

Yoga makes us sensitive to the language of the body. The physical body can say a lot about personality, and as you become attentive to your baby's style you learn a lot about who he is becoming. Dylan's optimistic nature was reflected in the ease of his body language. Rosey was physically confident and agile; she did a lot of backward arching, a reflection of her willful personality. Nissim dozed on his back like a starfish, as if he feared nothing; indeed, he turned into an outgoing physical daredevil. Uma, at five months, was scooting herself around the room far away from Mum, investigating every other baby. Mae was very peaceful and physically settled, mirroring her sanguine nature. Curious or cautious, flirtatious or reticent, it can often be read in babies' early body language.

The absence of competition in yoga class was one of the aspects of the practice that initially drew us to it, and we want to stress that Baby Om encourages a non-competitive atmosphere. The purpose of the baby engagement exercises is not to train the budding genius or the world-class athlete, although we have found through our teaching experience and conversations with mothers and child development experts that there are emotional as well as physical benefits that come along with this practice. For the infant, Baby Om offers a safe and nurturing environment and fosters growing confidence in movement and body awareness. The ability both to attach and then separate is achieved because the baby is involved in but is not the absolute focus of the mother's activity. Within this communication the baby has room to develop both connection and independence.

Another excellent benefit of this work is in fostering consciousness of how a parent cares for herself. A physically active parent presents an important role model and promotes continued participation in a child's future mental and physical health. You can think of this on a spectrum of activities that may later include participation in toddler gym classes, swimming, or skating.

Since a postpartum body is an ocean of change, and a new baby counts as one of life's major challenging events, yoga practice can be enjoyed for the unparalleled healing it can offer. Take the time, look within, grab your baby and your yoga mat, and begin sharing your life as a creative and healthy adult with the small wonder that has just arrived.

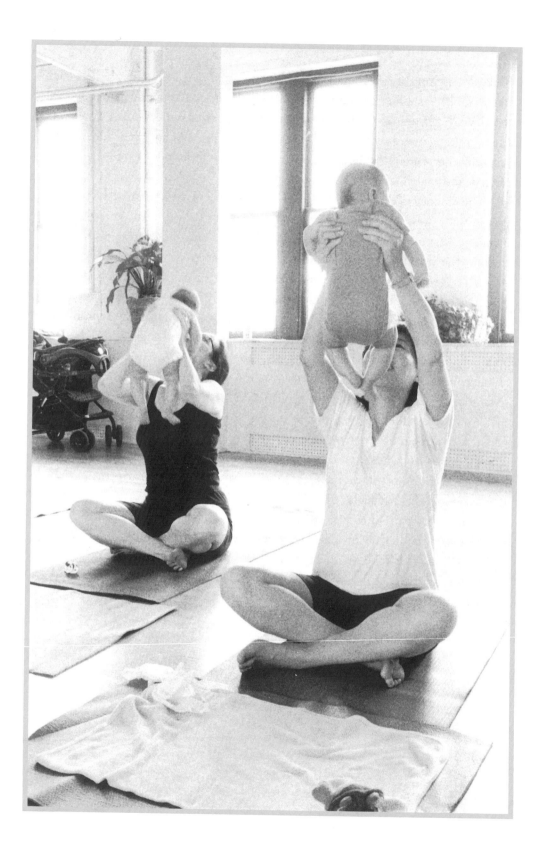

2

Baby Om Basics

This chapter presents the basics of Baby Om: when and where to practice, what to wear, and how to engage your baby. It provides a foundation for the four classes to follow. Remember, though, that these are only guidelines born of our experience—if a different approach feels better to you, feel free to try it.

Timing

First, when do you practice yoga? Initially, establishing a regular time will be hard—after all, as a new parent you'll be learning to grab time wherever you can find it. Ideally, it's good to set aside a "yoga hour" at approximately the same time each day. We all know that babies thrive on routine, and sometimes so do we; we rarely find time to do the many things we put off, especially when juggling the demands of an unpredictable baby. Whether you practice in the morning—fortifying yourself for the rest of the day—or plan your sessions for the afternoon lull, it helps to establish consistency in your timing. For many of us, yoga works best just after the baby's nap or feeding. We found that following Baby Om time, our babies were often either ready for a nap, or willing to spend a little time on their own, freeing up some quiet periods during which we felt fresh and rested. We also found that doing the class two to three times a week was just right, transforming our bodies and our enjoyment of our babies. Even if your practice is less frequent, you can enjoy the benefits of Baby Om.

Clothes

What you wear is another matter of preference. We suggest comfortable clothes that allow you to move freely. Our Baby Om standard uniform for the first year included black drawstring cotton pants, tank tops, and T-shirts. You don't need any special workout gear (unless you really love that kind of thing!). The baby, of course, need follow no dress code: whatever she can wiggle in is fine. We think "onesies" are great.

Environment and Equipment

Next, where to practice. All that's really required is a space at least the length of a yoga mat (1.8 meters or so) and the width of your arms spread out, fingers extended. The yoga mat itself, however, is almost a necessity (see Resources for where to find one; they are widely available from catalogs, online, and in bath product shops and chain stores). The mat prevents you from slipping while you are doing your poses, and pads the floor slightly. Babies seem to find the spongy rubber of sticky mats endlessly fascinating. That said, a hardwood floor is also acceptable, although you will want some kind of rug or padding to soften things up for your baby. In addition, you'll need at least one pillow; we prefer couch cushions over bed pillows. You will use this pillow to prop yourself up in certain positions (described in each class). Young babies also enjoy being propped up on their tummies, at the front of the mat, with extra pillows: it gives them security and develops their back extensor muscles while offering a new perspective on their stretching mum.

It is also worth finding a way to make your yoga time and space distinctive, by adding sounds, visuals, or scents that you feel will calm or otherwise enhance your practice. We often place candles, even scented unlit ones, in our space (lit candles should be far out of reach, of course). Sometimes we chant; sometimes we listen to music—any kind that adds to your relaxation will do and it doesn't even have to be officially "gentle." We've used Bach instrumentals and Schubert lieder, but also bossa nova, Janis Joplin, and Primal Scream.

Breathing

As in all yoga practices, an important basic to be aware of during your Baby Om sessions is your breathing. This is a fundamental aspect of yoga, and we'll return to it again and again in the classes. Try to use the first moments of each class to establish an awareness of your breath—the difficulty is sustaining the awareness, especially when you have a baby to contend with. However, breathing can be the best tool you have for discovering your natural rhythms, deepening your practice, and shedding anxiety. Paying attention to the quality of your breathing will make everything you do more effortless and deepen the effects of your practice. To do this, you will need to learn to become aware of your breath, which isn't as easy as it sounds. Standard yogic breathing involves inhaling and exhaling only through your nose. This may sound like what we do all our lives, but most people actually breathe through their mouths much of the time. One goal in the basic breathing exercise is to slow and deepen your breaths, making your inhalation exactly even (in count) with your exhalation. If your breath is shallow and fast, you are probably tightening your throat and abdominal area and not filling your full chest cavity. You may notice that you are breathing more in your "front body" and may need to focus your breath toward your "back body." A goal of breath awareness is to become more sensitive to your breathing patterns, and if this is experienced, it's a huge accomplishment.

Pre-*Asana* Breathing Practice (*Pranayama*)

Because of the natural delay in beginning *asana* practice, it is a good idea to practice the *pranayama* exercises first, which you can begin after about ten days. Keep the breath practices simple and set aside ten minutes where you lie down with a pillow underneath your back and head (to open your chest). Focus on steady exhalations and inhalations. Breathe in and out through your nostrils. When this feels comfortable you can add slight breath retention after each breath. You'll be amazed at how just this little exercise will restore you and clear your head.

Chanting

At the beginning and end of each class we usually chant *Om*, from one to three times, but this isn't mandatory. We do it because it marks the beginning and end of our practice, because it affects the body with the resonance of sound, and because the babies love it. To chant *Om*, let the sound rise up from your abdomen and release it through a relaxed and open throat. Give the same value to both the *o* and the *m*. Experiment with pitch and tone; some days your tone may be high, other days it might be low. We don't always hit the same note and the length is not always the same; regardless, the babies still perk up and take notice, and the feeling in the room changes as our energies become more unified.

Baby Exercises

The most important basic regarding the baby exercises is flexibility. Once you get a feel for these exercises, do as much or as little as you and your baby want, and select whatever mood feels right at the time, from stimulating play to soothing movement. Some days you may feel more focused on your child, others more on yourself: improvise and follow your instinct. Since each practice is a new experience for both of you—sometimes yielding unpredictable responses—we have found that the less of an agenda you set, the better. Never force your baby to do anything, but please note that a little fussing, especially when the baby is on her stomach (tummy play), is very common. Try to stay calm if your baby cries. Remember, a little frustration is considered beneficial for their future abilities in problem solving!

Moderation

This is vital: work carefully and steadily, especially at first. You probably won't have the same energy level that you had pre-pregnancy for quite a while, and you'll need to conserve and replenish the energy you do have. Remind yourself that yoga is not a race: the pace should be calm and measured rather than frenetic or strenuous. You don't need to force yourself to sit in the lotus position for an hour; nor do you need to attempt challenging or vigorous practice. There's no need to exhaust yourself (the baby will do that for you in any case). If you find yourself getting tired, slow down. Breathe more; do less. Remember, you just had a baby—you deserve a little rest!

Asana Guidelines

Last, a few guidelines that will inform your practice. This list was especially written with the postpartum body in mind. We know that this list won't answer all of your questions and that if you're a beginner some of this may sound complex, but we think these guidelines will give you enough information to see you through your postpartum year. Revisit this list throughout your Baby Om year. You'll find it all the more helpful.

1. When we talk about breaths we mean a full cycle of breathing that includes inhalation and exhalation.

2. Inhale and exhale through your nose. Your lips should stay relaxed.

3. Generally, you inhale in an upward or arching motion and exhale into a forward bending or downward one.

4. The more you can coordinate movement with breathing, the better and more internal your practice will be.

5. Always think about drawing the navel toward the spine (unless otherwise instructed) and lifting from the pubic bone to the navel. This slight contraction engages the lower abdominal muscles and pelvic floor and corrects a forward tilting pelvis. It will also help overtucking and/or overarching in the lower back.

6. Lifting of the pelvic floor, called *mula bandha* in yoga, is akin to the lifting action of Kegel exercises, which are suggested during pregnancy. An advanced practitioner keeps *mula bandha* lifted at all times throughout the practice. Notice the connection between lifting the pelvic floor and feeling lighter, alert, and energized.

7. Remember that your body is three-dimensional, with a front, back, and sides, which expands in all directions as you breathe. It is common to think only of the front and back, which can make your posture stiff, so keep this image in mind as you practice.

8. Lengthening the front of your thighs and lifting the hips will help your pelvis shift into a more vertical alignment after having been in a forward tilt for months during pregnancy. This will also help you stand up straighter.

9. Lift the front of your armpits higher than your back armpits; this will open the chest and lift breast tissue that may weigh down the chest. Sliding your shoulder blades down the spine will have a similar effect of lifting the chest. Another way to find this position is to stand with your arms loosely by your sides. Then rotate your hands so that your palms face front and then out to the side. Notice how your chest opens and your shoulder blades slide back and down.

10. Your arms, fingers included, should be relaxed and extended. Think of your arms as an extension of your heart.

11. The part of the body that contacts the floor (feet, hips, knees, hands) supports the weight of the body. Make sure that weight-bearing part is receptive and steady or your pose may feel unstable.

12. Pay special attention to your ankles and the alignment of your feet. The ankle ligaments may be overstretched, so be very aware of your ankle and foot placement. Imagine that there is an **X** on the sole of your foot and each complete line of the **X** has equal weight. When you do this, the ankle will become naturally aligned. Another image to try is to always keep the ankles stacked vertically over the heel, especially in wide-legged poses.

13. When the hands are weight-bearing (as in Downward Facing Dog) the fingers should be spread comfortably to support your weight. Your wrists should be parallel with the front of the mat and the middle fingers parallel to each other, and the pressure should be evenly distributed across the palm of the hand.

14. The rule for coming out of a pose is to retrace your steps. Come out of the pose the same way you went in to it.

15. Since you have spent the last nine months with your stance getting wider and wider, it will take time before it is comfortable to stand with your feet together again. We suggest you begin to work with your feet hip-width apart in *tadasana*, or Mountain Pose, for the first three months. Move them slightly closer for the

3–6-month class, and by six months, work with the feet either touching or up to two inches apart. Your pelvic structure has been affected by your pregnancy and it may take a long time, up to a year, for you to stand comfortably with your feet together. If this is true for you, work where it feels stable.

16. This is also true in Downward Facing Dog. You may start with your feet almost mat-width apart, and by 6–12 months, work with feet hip-width apart.

17. The opposite applies for wide-leg standing poses like Warrior I and II, Triangle, etc. Take the first six months to gradually widen your legs to the recommended 1.2 to 1.35 meters apart.

18. If your breasts are large or tender and make it difficult for you to do a pose (Lunge, for example), place your foot outside the hands (instead of *between* the hands) to create additional space. Other poses that may be affected by large or tender breasts are those done lying on your stomach. Place a pillow under your lower rib cage or rest on your forearms if you are uncomfortable.

19. If it hurts to sit on the floor due to hemorrhoids, an episiotomy, or a tear of the pelvic floor due to the birth process, sit on a pillow.

20. Yoga practice should be an addition to your life, not something punishing or something you feel compelled to do. Relax and enjoy!

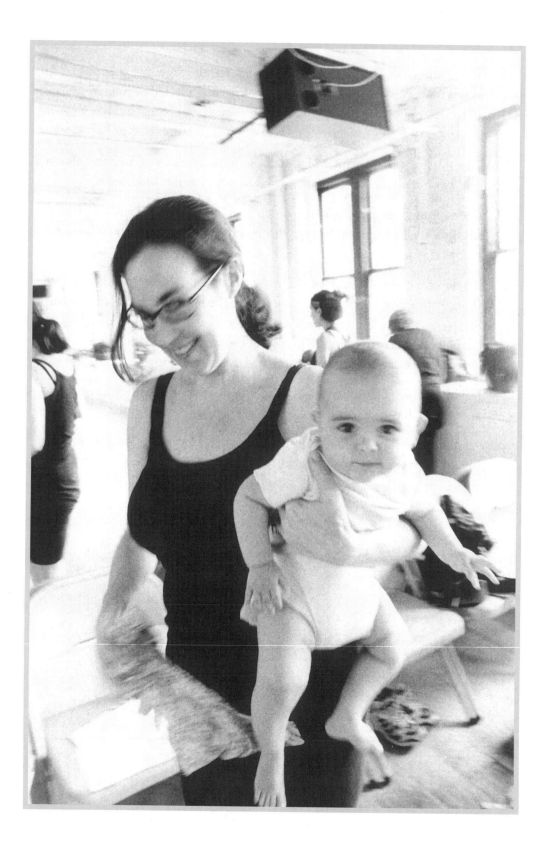

3

Baby Engagement

I n this chapter we tell you how you might approach this yoga playtime with your baby, especially if it's new to you. Getting your baby engaged, relaxed, and comfortable with this new form of play should be approached in a spirit of total acceptance and fun.

These exercises are a set of age-appropriate sequences, which we have included in each class. Some of the exercises may already be part of your baby play, and some may be completely new to you; either way, we will show you how we practice them. The exercises suggested are simple and easy to do. As far as baby interruptions go, take any time out that you need to nurse, comfort, or change your baby. This is all part of the experience of doing yoga with your infant. Try not to expect too much from baby or yourself. The improvisational aspect of Baby Om is the essence of this particular practice. We all start to recognize a pattern: babies act and caregivers react. There are no hard and fast rules for you as a pair in this practice.

When describing our baby engagement exercises, we illustrate our favorite ways to hold our babies' limbs. Don't rush the exercises—have fun and vary the timing, rhythm, and sounds or words you make. You'll find that infants respond well to soothing energy and an animated voice. Think of each exercise as a nursery rhyme—each one is contained and has its own pattern, structure, and sense of wholeness. We also suggest working with your baby's body in quadrants or parts—first the legs, then arms, then the whole body.

All of the Baby Om exercises can be done anytime and anywhere. (Many mothers tell us they use them to cheer up fussing babies.) The exercises you learn for a 0–3-month-old can still be done with a 3-, 6-, or even 12-month-old. As our babies grow we keep adding new exercises and new angles to old ones. This cumulative method gives infants a familiarity mixed with novelty that keeps them interested without becoming overstimulated.

Although Baby Om explores the developing relationship between caregiver and child, studies have shown that, much like adults, infants' motor pathways (or muscle memory) are improved by diligent repetition. If these exercises are done at the ages indicated, you can expect real benefits to your baby's coordination. So, even if you suspect you won't have the next Michael Jordan in your family, "the act of moving itself, especially when encouraged by an enthusiastic adult, does contribute to a child's ultimate success in physical activities," according to Lise Eliot, Ph.D., the author of *What's Going On in Here?* Babies are so thrilled by their own increasing coordination that it's worth the effort just to see their heart-melting joy.

Tummy play is typically part of each class, but the more time babies spend on their stomachs the better. When babies lie on their stomachs, they are subtly activating their front flexor muscles and strengthening their back and neck extensor muscles. Fairly quickly they learn to turn their heads from side to side and use their arms and hands to push against the floor as they develop the strength to lift their heads, involving themselves in their surroundings. The strength gained early on encourages the coordination of the limbs for quadrupedal locomotion (crawling). We firmly believe in the benefits of tummy play and urge mothers to begin it as early as possible. Our own children, Rosey and Miles, who loved being on their stomachs, turned out to be early crawlers. Bibi's daughter, Nina, was often completely serene and content—until she was placed on her stomach. Then Nina would become frustrated, but Bibi would stroke her back, telling her how much harder it was for mother than daughter. How true this is! Afterward, Nina would nurse a bit and become serene again. Now that babies are encouraged to sleep on their backs, tummy play is more important than ever.

We have also included in this chapter a few of our favorite age-appropriate exercises that are not necessarily done in each class, but that we love to do when we have the time, especially when it appears that the babies are on the cusp of learning a particular skill. Often the exercises will introduce and reinforce the mechanics of these movement skills, enough so that the babies really begin to integrate them into their bodies. We've often seen from our own kids that babies will learn a skill but their muscles will promptly forget it, perhaps not repeating the moment of adeptness again for several weeks. This is especially true when the movements require a lot of whole-body coordination, such as rolling over, crawling, kneeling, or walking. Just when you call your best friend to brag that your child has rolled over she won't do it again for the next two weeks. This would be a good time to practice the rolling exercise.

One last commonsense point: if your baby seems resistant, or works herself up into a real crying jag, don't force her to do the exercises. She may be hungry, tired, or just out of sorts. Try again tomorrow. Don't be put off if it takes her a few classes to fully relax in her new environment. It's not uncommon for the very young baby to fuss for the first few weeks and by her fourth month to have transformed into the biggest flirt in the class. We've seen it over and over, and by that point, of course, we're all in love!

Note from a Mum

Baby Om . . . such beautiful memories come to my mind. I started attending Baby Om classes when my son was three months old. I found it to be a supportive environment for both of us. Just the fact that everyone around me came also in "packages" of mother-and-baby was great but there was a lot more to it. Sarah and Laura were a wonderful teaching team—while one demonstrated an exercise, the other went around touching us to correct, stretch more, or give a little massage. Amazing how much comfort and energy a touch like that can give to a new mommy's heart. The yoga exercises were designed to fit "all sizes," so that even I, a nonathletic person, felt comfortable. I won't forget the feeling of one exercise, where we stretched our shoulders backward and opened the whole chest area . . . after holding and nursing a baby for almost three months straight . . . boy, did that feel good!

I would work out as much as my son had patience for, then nurse him, right there on the mat or alongside the wall, sitting next to another mummy-baby team that had to take a break. Sometimes my son actually fell asleep there. . . . Sarah and Laura also inspired me by bringing their own children to class. Going on with "adult" activities after having a baby, without leaving your baby behind, is so hard in our society, and it makes Baby Om a unique and wonderful experience. I would definitely do it again with my next baby.

— GALLIT, MOTHER OF ELI

A Confident Approach

As a general rule, you'll want to approach your baby with as much playfulness and tactile sensitivity as possible. We have seen some mothers who are so scared of hurting their newborns they can barely touch them, while others practically spin their babies around by one leg. Either way of relating is extreme. We remember being both surprised and impressed at how the OB nurses handled our newborns with such warm, matter-of-fact efficiency. If only we could learn such confidence, we felt.

Over time, we have. The more we experimented with our baby-play exercises, the more confident we became, especially when we saw how much Rosey and Dylan loved our attention and the security of our touch. Confidence in touch may come more naturally for some of you than others, but it is certainly something that can be learned. Playing with your baby is a universal language everyone can learn, and we will share some of the things we've discovered in our learning process.

Touch and Hold

When holding your baby in yoga class, make sure your fingers are relaxed and slightly spread, so that your hands span his rib cage. Keep your baby close to your center when you are standing and holding him. The more you support your baby while maintaining good alignment, by using your back and arms rather than your shoulders and neck, the stronger you'll feel (and become). Holding your baby too far away from your center puts an unhealthy strain on your back, neck, and shoulders.

Touch your baby the way you would want to be touched, firmly yet gently. You want to translate confidence to your baby, so be aware of yourself if you're feeling tentative. Infants are especially reactive to their environments because their nervous systems are still immature and becoming calibrated to life outside the womb. Loud noises and fast jerky movements startle them, and the same can be said for overly punctuated energy.

Massage

Babies really respond to massage. They learn to anticipate your touch and calm to it. Although professional technique is not required, there are certain simple massage skills that are easy to learn and follow the natural functions of the body. For example, when massaging your baby's arms and legs, stroke them in an outward motion to encourage limb extension. When massaging the stomach, move in a clockwise motion beginning at the lower right quadrant, just above the right leg. This motion follows the movement of the digestive tract. When massaging the back, stroke downward from the shoulders to the hips and also from the spine around to the front of the rib cage when the baby is on his side. Pay special attention to the soles of the feet and palms of the hands, especially in the first three months. If you cannot fit massage into each class, try making it part of your after-bath, diaper-change, or pre-bedtime ritual. Massage is especially important for pre-term babies.

Swinging, Turning, and Moving in Space (3–12 Months)

These exercises are for infants who have established good head control. Babies love moving in space and this can be a welcome break in the middle of class. Your baby will be secure in your arms, and you will be performing a duet. Whether your baby prefers facing inward or outward doesn't matter; the exciting effect of movement will be the same. The internal system affected by these exercises is the one that later on deals with your baby's balance and postural control, knowing where she is in space and in relation to gravity (vestibular system).

Note from a Mum

Baby Om, like any activity you attempt with a new baby, is a process. Be patient and stick with it. The first attempts at exercising are hard, and synchronizing the right time, place, and mood with an infant is nearly impossible. However, over time it gets easier and it is well worth the effort. I can now confidently say the Baby Om classes have been a lifesaver for me. Not only have they allowed me a way to reconnect with my body, but they have also provided my daughter and me with a regular playdate and have taught us a language of movement that we have made our own and do several times a day. It makes us happy.

— MARI, MOTHER OF ZOE

BABY ENGAGEMENT EXERCISES

SQUEEZE HOLD
0–3 MONTHS

This exercise is especially good for bringing proprioceptive (sensory) awareness to the newborn's joints. Starting at either the hip or shoulder joints, encircle your baby's joint and limb with your hands. Moving down the arms and legs, squeeze and release, giving even, gentle pressure to the entire circumference of your hand. Think about how you might check for ripeness in a fruit. Work on each joint in succession.

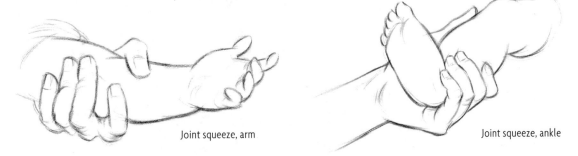

Joint squeeze, arm

Joint squeeze, ankle

KNUCKLE RUB
0–3 MONTHS

Grasping is a hand movement that actually begins when the baby is still in utero. It is considered a reflexive movement until about the age of three months when the baby begins to differentiate hand from arm. To help release your newborn's clenched fingers, rub the backs of his fingers together and they will gradually relax and extend.

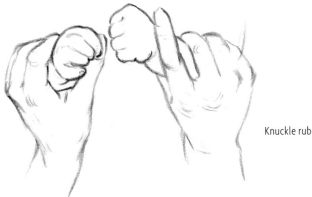

Knuckle rub

SPINE STROKE

0–3 MONTHS

This exercise will stimulate the back and neck muscles and the feeling of the mat on the baby's belly will give him important sensory information. Place your baby on his tummy. Use one of your fingers to gently stroke the length of his spine from the back of his neck to his tailbone. This encourages a back arch and head lift.

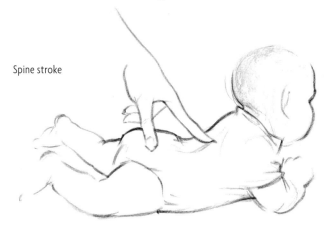

Spine stroke

HANDS ON THE FLOOR

0–6 MONTHS

This exercise develops your baby's awareness of pressing into and pushing away from the floor. It is great for upper-body strength and pre-crawling. With your baby lying on her tummy, attempt to uncurl her fingers and place her open palms on the floor. Press her palms gently down and allow the hands to get used to feeling the surface of the floor.

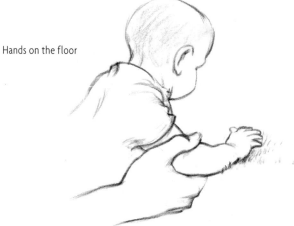

Hands on the floor

SOLES OF FEET TOGETHER

0–6 MONTHS

This gives your baby tummy time while stimulating the proprioceptors (sensory neurons) on the soles of the foot. The legs and feet are the last body parts to "motorically mature," and this is a great pre–weight-bearing exercise. With your baby lying on her tummy, pat and rub the soles of her feet together.

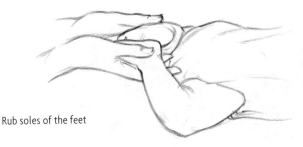

Rub soles of the feet

FEET ON THE FLOOR

3–6 MONTHS

Although your baby is far too young to support any of his own weight in a standing posture, help him practice placing the soles of his feet evenly on the floor as you support him in an upright position. This will help him begin to extend through the legs and uncurl his toes after nine months in a fetal curl.

Feet on the floor

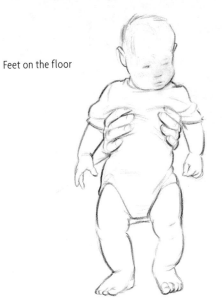

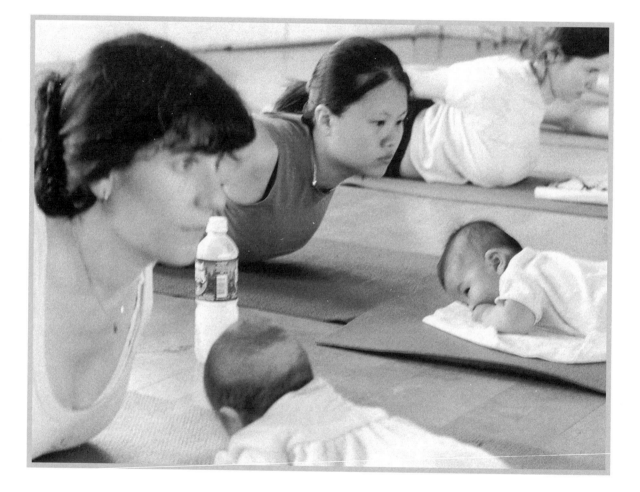

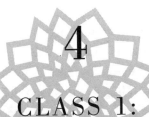

4

CLASS 1:
The First Three Months

A CLASS FOR SOOTHING AND QUIETING
APPROXIMATELY 30 MINUTES; HOLD EACH POSE FOR THREE TO FIVE BREATHS.

Sounded Breath

Star Pose

Sun Salute, Series 1

Plank Pose

Standing Forward Bend

Lunge

Mountain Pose

Tree Pose

Warrior II

Triangle Pose

Head to Knee Pose

Modified Boat Pose

Locust Pose

Half Wheel Pose

Sage Pose

Seated Forward Bend

Resting Pose

Much has been written and filmed about the joy a new baby brings to our lives. Although that is certainly true, those early months with a newborn can also be a time of extreme emotions from both ends of the spectrum. Childbirth is a dramatic, demanding event calling upon all our physical and emotional resources. And then there is a new life to care for and bond with.

No two birthing stories are ever alike. Each birth has its own physical and mental aftermath. We've worked with mothers whose births went exactly as they imagined they would and those for whom childbirth took unexpected turns. Your mother's or your sister's delivery experience may have been quick and straightforward, while you were in labor for what seemed like three days. You planned to take painkillers and ended up barely making it to the hospital before your baby was born.

Whatever your story, your baby has finally arrived. You did it! Congratulations! You are a parent now and you have a heart-melting infant who will change your life forever. With your infant's birth still fresh in your memory your life as a mum has begun. Your son or daughter is here waiting to learn all about the world from you. Things you've seen many times suddenly seem new: if it's winter, the air has never been crisper; if it's summer the sun was never as golden. Birth is only one small part of becoming a parent, and only the beginning of the process of raising a child.

With the new routine of taking care of a newborn to get used to, a simple trip to the market seems like mounting an Everest expedition. Never mind remembering to pack the diaper bag with three diapers, two pacifiers, a box of wipes, tissues, a cloth diaper (for spit-ups), and an extra set of clothes for baby. When all these details begin to feel oppressive, keep in mind that you will miss this phase of your baby's life when it is behind you. It's a time that seems as if it will last forever but ends with great finality.

This is a time of immense change and we want to help make this transition as smooth as possible. We know that in these early months, you may be subjected to a barrage of well-intended advice from everyone from your mother to total strangers. Somehow everyone knows more about you and your baby than you do. Is it possible? You get unsolicited advice from all sides about feeding, dressing, bathing, and holding your baby. Some friends suggest that you return to work as soon as you can, while others advise you to steer clear of the workplace for the next fifteen years.

While those around you may wish for a new job or a boyfriend, those desires pale in comparison to your own wish for a full night's sleep—an unimaginable luxury.

During this period, doing yoga might not be the first thing on your mind, but whether you are running on adrenaline or exhaustion, the restorative aspect of yoga will definitely help you feel better and may be just what you need.

Note from a Mum

Baby Om is a great way to get back in shape and have a fun, relaxing time to bond with your baby, whether she or he is a newborn, a toddler, or anywhere in between. You feel that you're doing something wonderful for your body, your mind, and your baby. My son Ben loves it as much as I do!

— AMY, MOTHER OF BEN

The Class

Considering the many demands that are being made on you in the first three months of your baby's life, this is a time when you don't want to deplete your energy. The *asanas* in Class 1 have been selected for their soothing and gentle energizing qualities. The class begins with a series of poses to open the chest, relieving tight muscles in the upper back, neck, and shoulders which are often related to carrying and nursing your baby. The standing poses work on leg strength, endurance, and alignment of the whole body. Plank Pose and Downward Facing Dog strengthen the arm and shoulder area. Modified Boat Pose and the Half Wheel series challenge and build much-needed abdominal stamina. Twists, such as Head to Knee Pose, tone and bring fresh blood to the internal and reproductive organs that have been compromised as your baby grew and shifted position inside you. Hip openers will help to rebalance the symmetry of the pelvis.

The restorative qualities of each of these poses will nourish your energy and relieve exhaustion. You must wait for the lochia (postpartum bleeding) to stop before beginning Class 1, although a little discharge is okay. This can take anywhere from two to six weeks, but generally women are ready by the third or fourth week. If you begin bleeding again after going through a class it is a sign you have done too much and should cut back to the breathing exercises.

The waiting period between your baby's birth and when you begin your practice is the perfect time to work on some basic breathing and Kegel exercises, as it is essential to strengthen the pelvic floor before adding intraabdominal pressure from other abdominal exercises. Something as simple as making your inhalation and exhalation of even duration can make you feel grounded and refreshed. The *pranayama*, or breathing technique, we recommend for this interval can be found on page 39. You should certainly practice Kegel exercises (tightening the pelvic floor in any position), also called in yoga terms *mula bandha*, or root lock. See chapter 10 for an in-depth discussion of Kegels. Also, lie on the floor with your knees bent and practice drawing your navel inward toward your spine as you exhale, engaging your abdominal muscles. If you are new to yoga or if you feel this class is too challenging, we suggest you practice the C-section class (see chapter 7) until you are ready to move on. At the end of the three-month period, don't feel that you must move on to Class 2 if you are not quite ready. Continue with Class 1 or alternate with the cesarean class.

Your Body

During the three months following the birth of your baby, your body is slowly returning to its pre-pregnancy state. You may feel exhausted, and your former self may seem either like a lost acquaintance you barely remember or one you remember all too well, if only because every article of clothing in your closet reminds you of her. Your breasts may seem huge and out of control; you may have veins like a map. Sarah recalls the added insult of still having to wear her maternity clothes. It is a time when your self-image may be temporarily turned upside down, and as one new mother said, the four scariest words in the English language are: "Bring your bathing suit." Later, you may not even recognize yourself in photographs, as Laura didn't when she saw a picture of herself taken at a party five weeks after she had given birth. Women have tried all kinds of schemes, from crash diets to avoiding breast-feeding, in order to lose weight. Even if you've lost much of the pregnancy weight, you're still carrying extra kilos and centimeters, depending on your eating habits, physical activity, and whether or not you nurse.

Some women feel great after giving birth, while others are reminded of the event every time they move for the next three months. Wherever you fall in this range of experience, it's a good idea to start slowly, bearing in mind all the changes your body has gone through. Don't look in the closet, dwelling on all the clothing you can't wait to wear. Recovery is a process. You will get there completely or partially, but whatever the outcome, you have a fabulous baby and you will be bending, literally, to meet his needs as well as your own. The physical aspect of life after birth is full of adjustments.

Before you begin yoga we want you to be aware of some postpartum basics. But first, a quick anatomy lesson is in order. Muscles hold the skeleton in place. Tendons are the ends of muscles. Tendons attach to the bone and act as levers. Ligaments attach bone to bone and act as beams. Ligaments have less blood flow than tendons. Pregnancy makes all the ligaments of your body more flexible due to an infusion of the hormones progesterone and relaxin. Ligaments aren't elastic structures, so if you overstretch them, they don't readily bounce back. This can result in permanently unstable joints: ligaments of the pelvis, symphysis pubis (pubic bone), sacrum, and hips can be particularly susceptible after the birthing process. You need to make your muscles strong again to support the joints. Never overwork your joints. If you have *any* joint pain, stop working immediately.

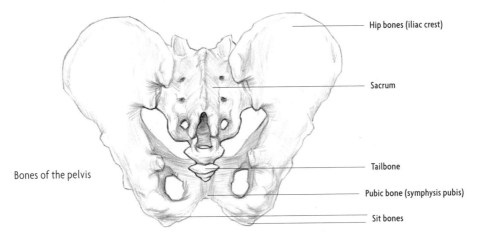

Hip bones (iliac crest)

Sacrum

Bones of the pelvis

Tailbone

Pubic bone (symphysis pubis)

Sit bones

The pelvic area has certain boney "landmarks" we mention when describing the poses (see illustration). We refer to the *sit bones* frequently. These are the boney protrusions on the bottom of your pelvis. You can feel them if you sit in a cross-legged position and rock your pelvis forward and backward. We also make reference to the sacrum, which is the bony triangle at the bottom of the spine that connects the two halves of the pelvis and consists of five naturally fused vertebrae. Below the sacrum is the tailbone, three more fused vertebrae that generally curve slightly in toward the front of the body. The sacrum and the tailbone form the bottom of your spine. You might think of the sacrum as a plant bulb and the spine as the emerging green stem.

For an in-depth discussion of the physical effects of pregnancy and childbirth, see chapter 11 for postpartum conditions. If you know, for instance, that you have pregnancy-related carpal tunnel syndrome, we include additional suggestions for how and when to practice yoga.

Besides a feeling of overall weakness, you may possibly experience edema (swelling) of the lower legs; tightness in the upper back, neck, and sacrum; diastasis (separation of the abdominal wall); sciatica; and pain around the sacrum and hips. You may be recovering from an episiotomy or natural tear in the pelvic floor. These are complaints, some minor, some less so, that we've seen over and over in our classes. The conditions do improve over time.

Your center of balance shifted when you were pregnant; the weight of your baby pulled your center line so that it fell not over the arch of your feet but in front of your toes. Normally, this plumb line extends from the top of your head to your feet, with your ears directly over your shoulders, and your hips balanced evenly over your knees and these over your ankles. This imaginary vertical line doesn't auto-matically snap back after birth. Imagine a vertical line of building blocks in which a few of the blocks have shifted, throwing the column off.

An across-the-board problem we've encountered is lower-back pain, due pri-marily to all the stooping and lifting inherent in the tasks of motherhood. Between changing diapers, bending over strollers, carrying the weight of a baby in a front or backpack carrier, and maybe even lifting other young siblings, standing up straight can become a challenging activity. The poses in this class will address this. Regain-ing strength in your abdominal muscles will help support your back. Also, get in the habit of bending your knees when you pick up your baby. Regrettably, we didn't, and had to train ourselves months later as we started to suffer back pain from lugging around what were now our very heavy babies. Remember that repetitive movements such as lifting, holding, and feeding also contribute to pain and strain.

Fatigue and spaciness at this point in time can be overwhelming, but you will find that doing anything physical will improve not just your circulation and respiration, but your outlook as well. This is especially important if you are experiencing postpartum depression (see chapter 9). Remember that this is a period of sweeping transition for new mothers. You now have the needs of two, rather than one relatively free agent, to contend with. The sense of responsibility is huge and can be overwhelming.

If just reading this description of possible problems makes you feel like a woman on the verge of total collapse, take a deep breath, but don't give up. The litany of potential postpartum *conditions* may make you feel overwhelmed, but the fact is, bones will realign and muscles will regain their tone with a little effort in the right direction.

Your Baby

The first three months is the period that many people consider to be the fourth trimester for both mother and baby. It's a time of enormous growth, development, and adjustment for all concerned. During the first three months of life, your baby is working on three primary skill sets. The most important one is the ability to bond with his caregivers. The second is the development of vision, and third is head and neck control. You will be astonished at how much your baby changes over these three months.

During the first weeks of life, babies often resemble little frogs, with their knees tucked way up on either side of their chests. Their limbs are held close to their bodies and their hands curled into tight little fists. Their movements tend to be jerky, as if startled. Babies are born with five major innate reflexes that help them thrive and grow and gradually develop into active physical patterns. Some of the reflexes are protective, such as sucking, rooting, and grasping, and the other two—the Moro (startle) and the Babinski (toe-stretching) reflexes—are more reactive. We remember our husbands shrieking, pale from pain, as the babies grabbed handfuls of their chest hair and their tiny fingers had to be gently pried open.

Infants get the majority of their stimulation visually and they start life able to focus on objects 20 to 25 centimeters away, about the distance from breast to face.

Objects with high definition, like the human face, sun-drenched windows, and brightly colored objects stand out, while things too near or in the distance remain blurry. At around eight weeks they can track moving objects with their eyes, and though they may break eye contact with people, they are able to reconnect a few moments later. The transformation to near-adult vision occurs at about four to six months, so bear in mind that just practicing yoga near your baby during these early weeks provides a huge amount of essential stimuli and information. You will want to maintain gentle and playful eye contact, and as your baby grows you can experiment with having him follow your hands, arms, and gaze.

At around three months babies begin to bend and stretch their arms and legs, extending their limbs in space. Their fingers can now uncurl, and they can occasionally rest a flat open palm on your chest while nursing. They begin to bat and hold objects in their hands for short periods of time as they develop the fine motor skills that develop into the pincer grip, generally around nine months of age. The muscles of their torso begin to develop enough so they can recline in a supported sitting position, and they can generally control head movement.

An infant's nervous system is sensitive and easily overstimulated. Babies like to be held, often in an upright position, and are soothed by rocking. Your baby may not yet have a consistent daily routine and will spontaneously fall asleep at odd times, so don't expect her always to stay awake throughout your practice. During her home practice, Laura's son Miles would often fall into a deep peaceful sleep midway through the *asanas*. Babies in this age group are also beginning to make sounds of contentment when feeding and are starting to communicate with little barks and coos—the first signs of language. One of the biggest developmental delights occurs when your baby begins to smile at you and actively returns your smile.

The exercises in this 0–3-month class are designed especially to engage basic motor functions. They promote extension of the baby's limbs through simple leg and arm movements, and relaxation of contracted muscles by gently wiggling the limbs. Through range-of-motion and simple joint rotation exercises your baby will be encouraged to move her arms and legs independently and develop gross muscular coordination. We also suggest gentle baby massage concentrating on the palms of the hands and soles of the feet, which helps bring basic sensory awareness to these areas.

BREATHING EXERCISE FOR 0–3 MONTHS:
SOUNDED BREATH

We recommend this breath not only for the pre-*asana* practice but also for any time of stress. It's a basic breath that's useful for slowing down and calming the nervous system. You can do this in a sitting or reclining position, while you are nursing, or quietly on your own.

- Sit in a comfortable cross-legged position on a cushion, or recline with a cushion under your chest and head.
- Let your downward gaze be softly unfocused (as if you could see inside and outside yourself at the same time) or close your eyes lightly.
- Release your jaw and the muscles of your face (your teeth should be parted).
- Let that same sense of release move down your body, neck, shoulders, chest, etc.
- Inhale and exhale evenly through your nose, but try to draw the breath from down in your throat. Your throat and jaw should stay relaxed.
- Continue to breathe in this way, with the sound audible only to you. The sound may be like whispered waves along the shore.
- As you inhale, be aware of the belly and chest expanding evenly in all directions at once.
- As you exhale, keep the chest open and lifted (don't collapse).
- Allow your relaxation to slow your breath. Repeat ten times.

STAR POSE (*Tarasana*)

Mum
- Begin in a seated position with the soles of your feet together about 45 centimeters in front of your hips.
- Draw your sit bones evenly into the floor.
- Bend forward from the hips and walk your arms out beyond your feet and baby, moving your head toward your feet.
- Keep the spine long and extended and shoulders relaxed, shoulder blades moving down the back.

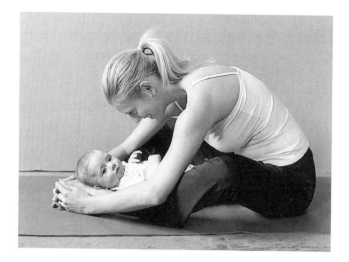

Star Pose

- Relax the abdomen and breathe into the full length and width of your back.
- Once you have established your pose, chant *Om* to your baby.
- After you have finished your *Om*(s), practice your Kegels five to ten times.

Baby

- Rest your baby's head in the soles of your feet. Gaze into her eyes as you release into the stretch, getting closer and closer.
- Hold her to your chest, supporting her head while you "circle your spine."

Essentials

Remember that this is a preliminary stretch, so don't push. Breathe into it.

What if . . .

If you feel you can't come forward, sit on a pillow and move your feet farther from your hips.

Cool Thing

This pose feels so great to do. Your baby is the *star* of the pose as she tempts you forward.

Variation for Back and Hips

- After the forward bend (see page 52), sit up straight and rotate your torso in a circle; imagine that you are drawing circles on the ceiling with the top of your head. Circle first in one direction, then the other.

Variation to Open Chest

- Sit in Star Pose.
- Interlace your fingers behind your back with the palms together.
- Press the knuckles into the floor and lift the chest, rolling the upper arms outward, away from the heart.
- Change the cross of your fingers and repeat.

BABY ENGAGEMENT IN TARASANA

*T*arasana engagement exercises are a wonderful way to begin class. Immediately, they involve your baby in your practice and your baby becomes secure in your attention. You are slowly starting to warm up your body and your baby is discovering her own through your guidance and touch. Generally we begin with baby squeezes, then move through the legs, arms, and the whole torso. Experiment, be silly, have fun.

Mum

If sitting comfortably in Star Pose is hard, try a cross-legged position or wide-leg pose.

Baby

Your baby is on her back, feet toward you. If you are in Star Pose (soles of feet together) her head will rest between your feet, or sit cross-legged.

Pressure Squeezes

Gently but firmly squeeze each of your baby's joints in succession, from the center of her body outward (see illustration on page 27).

- Start from each shoulder and work through the elbow, forearm, and wrist, ending with the palm and through to each fingertip. Then give a few smooth strokes to her palm.

- Do the same with your baby's hips, knees, ankles, and the sole of each foot through to the tips of the toes. End with a few long strokes from heel to toe on the sole of her foot.

For Baby's Lower Body

- Holding your baby's lower legs, press his knees toward his chest and then extend the legs as you feel returned pressure. Repeat five times.
- Bicycle the baby's legs in toward his chest one at a time, alternating sides. Repeat five times for each leg.
- With both of his knees in toward his chest, rock your baby side to side. Repeat five times to each side.

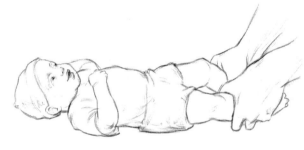

Hands holding baby's legs—legs long

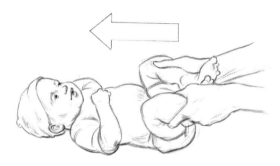

Hands holding baby's legs—knees to chest

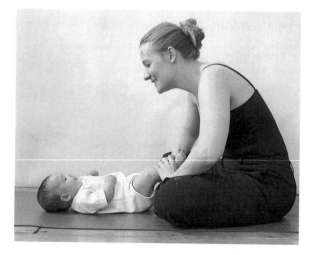

Baby's legs with mother holding legs down

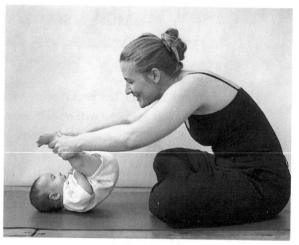

Baby's legs with feet to head

- Place fingertips of both your hands under his sacrum or mid-diaper, and gently bounce him.
- Hold his ankles and gently move his feet toward his forehead, rolling up and down along his spine (see photos, page 42). Repeat three to five times.

For Baby's Upper Body

- Holding your baby's hands in your own, slowly bring them across her chest.
- Gently open them to her sides. If you feel resistance give a gentle wiggle and repeat.
- Do this in an easy rhythm, keeping it simple, but as your baby grows (over a matter of weeks) add clapping and rhythmic variation like open and clap, and open and clap.
- Start with one arm reaching gently overhead. Move the arm around in a wide circle ending by her side. Repeat on the other side.
- Circle the baby's hands around each other in front of her chest, first one way and then the other (as in the song, "The Wheels on the Bus Go 'Round and 'Round . . .").

Massage

- Slowly stroke from the baby's shoulders down to her hips.
- Place your thumbs together at the center of your baby's chest and stroke outward toward her arms and hands.

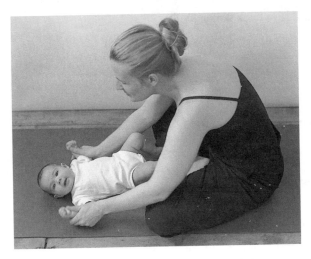

Baby's arms open

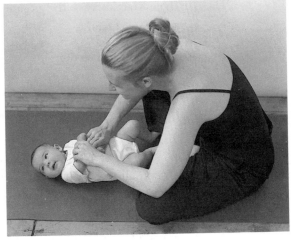

Baby's arms closed

- Using long strokes, massage from the hips down through calves, ankles, and feet.
- Massage her face with your thumbs, outward from nose to ears.

SUN SALUTE, SERIES 1 *(Surya Namaskar)*

There are many versions of the Sun Salute, a flowing sequence of poses often used to begin yoga classes. It warms up the body and stimulates circulation. This series uses the following poses.

Cat and Cow
- Start on all fours in the neutral Cat and Cow position.
- Move in and out of the pose, inhaling into Cow and exhaling into Cat. Repeat a few times.

Downward Facing Dog *(Adho Mukha Svanasana)*
- Exhale into the position.
- Remain there for three breaths.

Child's Pose *(Balasana)*
- Exhale, your knees to the ground and hips back to the heels.
- Stay for two breaths.

Repeat the sequence three times.

CAT AND COW

Mum
- Begin on all fours, with your shoulders over your wrists and your hips over your knees.
- Keep your weight evenly distributed between the hands and the knees.
- Draw your navel slightly in toward the spine, engaging the abdominal muscles.

- Spread your fingers apart and put weight into the knuckles as well as the palms of your hands, as if to press the floor away. Your fingers will point forward, with the middle fingers of each hand parallel.
- Broaden across your chest, allowing your shoulder blades to move down the back.
- As you inhale slowly, arch your back, bringing the tailbone and head up toward the ceiling (Cow stretch).
- As you exhale slowly, reverse the posture, rounding the back and bringing the tailbone and head down toward the floor with the navel drawn toward the spine (Cat stretch). Repeat three to five times.

Baby

Your baby is lying on the mat with her head directly below your head. She may reach for your face and hair; she is doing "pre-reaching," paving the way for her hand-eye coordination.

Essentials

Keep the movement fluid as you do this pose. You are warming up as you glide from Cow to Cat and back.

What if . . .

If your knees hurt on the floor, place a folded blanket under them for padding.

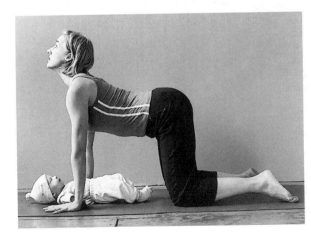

Cow Pose

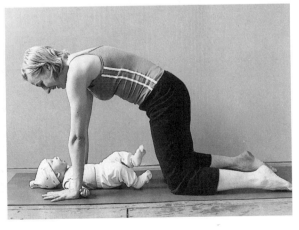

Cat Pose

Cool Thing

Your baby will love your movement and proximity.

Variation to Release the Lower Back

- Start on hands and knees, as in the previous instructions.
- Rock backward with your hips toward your heels then forward, letting your chest move out over your baby, your shoulders over your wrists.
- Inhale as you move forward and exhale as you move back. Repeat three times in each direction.

DOWNWARD FACING DOG *(Adho Mukha Svanasana)*

Mum

- Start in Cat and Cow neutral position (neither arched nor rounded).
- With your fingers spread wide, distribute the weight evenly throughout your hands.
- Spread your feet apart almost to mat width. Tuck your toes under and float your hips toward the ceiling.
- Straighten your legs, move your thighs back, and lift the kneecaps.

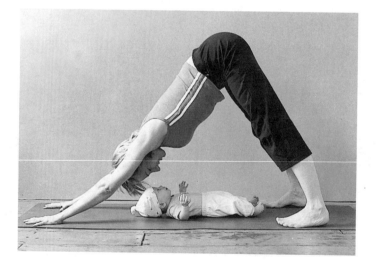

Downward Facing Dog

- Reach down and back with your heels and stretch your toes forward.
- Press and lengthen from the hands through the spine to the sit bones, making one long diagonal line.
- Draw the lower abdomen in toward the spine.
- Release your head and neck, letting it drop slightly toward your baby.

Baby

Your baby is lying on the mat directly below your chest, resting so that you meet eye to eye when in the pose. Say hello as you move into the position.

Essentials

Extend from the palms of the hands to the pelvis, thinking of the sit bones as the high point of the pose.

What if . . .

If your spine is unable to extend, bend your knees slightly and try again to lengthen the spine by lifting the pelvis toward the ceiling.

Cool Thing

You are one step closer to doing future handstands in the park with your child. (Downward Facing Dog contains the fundamentals of the handstand.)

CHILD'S POSE *(Balasana)*

Mum

- Kneel with the tops of your feet on the floor, your toes touching and your knees apart.
- Bend forward, creasing at the hips. Your hips should remain resting on your heels, with the sit bones pointing down.
- Walk your arms out in front of you to rest your torso comfortably along your upper legs.
- Relax your abdomen and broaden across the lower back.

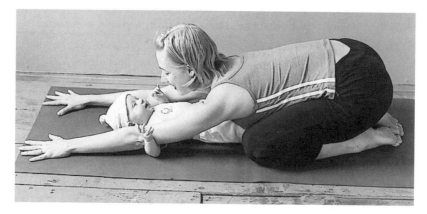

Child's Pose

Baby

Your baby is lying face up on the floor between your knees so you can kiss and cuddle with her as you rest in the pose.

Essentials

This is a restorative pose, so breathe deeply and release into it.

What if . . .

If you feel as if you're falling forward, place your elbows on either side of your baby and give a little pressure backward toward the sit bones.

Cool Thing

This is a great opportunity to release residual tension in the belly. Relax and play peek-a-boo with your baby.

Variation to Stretch Your Feet

- Start by kneeling, with your toes tucked under so that you are stretching the "neck" of the toes.
- Keep your inner ankles and calves together. Sit on your heels to deepen the stretch.
- Stay for a few breaths, then release.

PLANK POSE

Mum

- Start in Downward Facing Dog.
- Move your body forward until your shoulders are over the wrists.
- Make one long, extended line from your head to your heels.
- Keep your arms straight, with the inner elbows rolled forward.
- Look slightly ahead of you at your baby on the floor.
- Keep your shins and thighs lifted and the tailbone pointing toward the heels.
- Broaden your collarbone and move the shoulder blades slightly together.
- Draw the navel toward the spine, imagining that you are wrapping from the sides of your waist to your midline.
- Hold for one to three breaths, then move back into Downward Facing Dog.

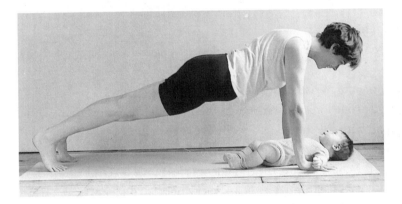

Plank Pose

Baby

Your baby is lying on the mat between your hands. For the variation she is lying between your forearms.

Essentials

Keep your arms very straight, revolving the inner elbows forward.

What if . . .

If you feel discomfort in the lower back, you might be sagging in the hips. Work on connecting to your center by lengthening your tailbone toward the heels, keeping your legs straight, heels pulling back and abdominal muscles firm.

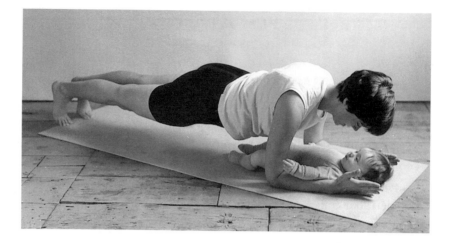

Elbow Plank

Cool Thing
Imagine you can levitate while you work on strengthening the whole body.

Variation for Wrist Pain (Elbow Plank)
- Place your forearms on the ground, parallel to each other, shoulder-width apart with the shoulders directly above the elbows.
- Your hands are on either side of your baby, palms facing in.
- Lift the chest, letting the shoulder blades move together down the back.
- With your feet hip-width apart, tuck your toes under, straighten the legs, and lift your knees off the mat.
- Keep the hips in line with the body, creating a straight line.
- Draw the navel up and in, engaging the abdominal muscles.
- Remain here for one to three breaths.

Side Plank Variation
- Start in Plank Pose.
- Bend your left leg so that the knee and shin are fully on the mat and parallel to its front edge.
- Place the inside edge of your right foot on the mat in line with your left hand.

- Rest your weight on the right leg, which is very straight, and left shin, which is on the mat.
- Turn your body to face the side; make one extended line from your foot to your head.
- Reach your right hand to the ceiling, stacking the right shoulder directly over the left.
- Make sure that the elbow of the supporting arm is not hyperextended. If it is, relax the joint by bending it slightly.
- Keep your hips lifted and chest open, with your navel drawn toward the spine.
- To change sides extend the bottom leg to meet the top leg, then shift back to Plank Pose.
- Rest between sides.

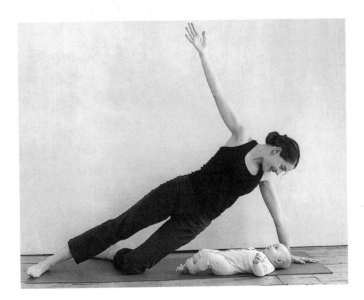

Side Plank Variation

STANDING FORWARD BEND (*Uttanasana*)

Mum

- Stand with your feet about hip-width apart or slightly wider.
- Bend forward from the hips, keeping your legs straight and kneecaps lifted, engaging the muscles of the thighs.
- Widen and release the lower back.
- Feel the heels pulling to the ground and the sit bones to the ceiling.
- Keep the feet, especially the toes, relaxed, and spread wide.
- Imagine your torso spilling over from the pelvic area like water.
- With every breath, release a little farther toward the mat.
- Drop your head toward your feet.

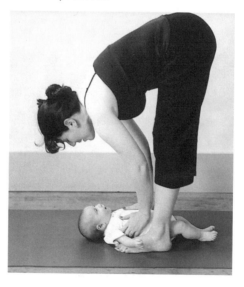

Standing Forward Bend

Baby

Your baby is lying between your feet on the mat. You can give her a squeeze and rock her side-to-side with the insides of your ankles. As your upper body pours toward the mat, you can easily hold her hands. Look into her eyes as she draws you forward.

Essentials

Keep the sit bones directly over the heels.

What if . . .

If your hamstrings or lower back feel very tight, let your knees bend slightly.

Cool Thing

This inverted pose is very calming to the nervous system.

Variation for Warming Hamstrings and Back

- From the Forward Bend, inhale and extend your spine, lifting your upper body until it is parallel to the mat. Keep your back flat.
- Draw the navel toward the spine.
- Keep the hips over the heels.
- Hold your baby's hands.
- Exhale and fold back down toward the mat. Repeat.

LUNGE *(with a straight leg)*

Mum

- Start in Forward Bend with your feet about hip-width apart.
- Bend your knees until your fingertips can touch the floor on the outside of your feet.
- Reach your right leg straight back as far as is comfortable.
- Your left knee should be directly over the left heel, and you should be able to see your left toes. Adjust as needed to achieve this.
- Stretch your right heel back, straightening the right knee, and enjoy the stretch for the front of your back leg.
- Keep your hips even and parallel to the floor.
- Lengthen your spine and broaden your collarbones, rising up on your fingertips to open the chest and allow the shoulder blades to move slightly down the back and toward each other.
- To come out of it bring the back foot forward to the starting position.
- Repeat, bringing the left leg back.

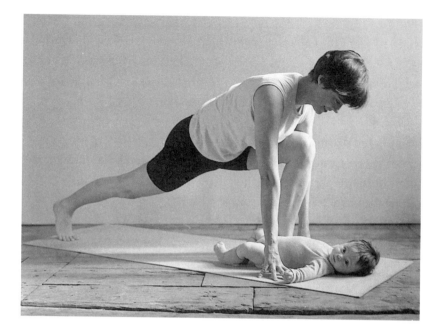

Lunge (with a straight leg)

Baby

Your baby is on the mat between your feet.

Essentials

Draw the navel up and in to allow your abdominals to support the position.

What if . . .

If the stretch feels too intense for the front of your thigh or if it is too hard to hold, let your back knee rest on the floor and let the hips move back into a more comfortable stretch.

Cool Thing

This is a great stretch to open and extend the front of the hip and thigh. Remind yourself to lift your abdominal organs.

MOUNTAIN POSE *(Tadasana)*

Mum

- Stand with your feet hip-width apart and your arms down alongside the body, middle finger touching about mid-thigh.
- Imagine a plumb line extending from the top of your head to between your ankles.
- Balance the weight evenly between the front and back of the feet.
- Lift your kneecaps and your thigh muscles, engaging the quadriceps.
- Allow your head to float above your shoulders.
- Broaden the collarbones and allow your shoulder blades to move slightly together and down your back.
- Draw your navel up and in.

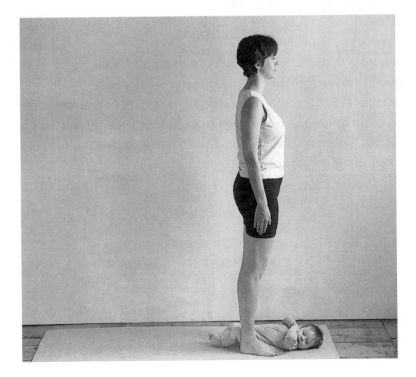

Mountain Pose

Baby

Your baby is on the mat between your feet if they are hip-width apart, or in front of you if your ankles are together.

Essentials

When rolling into and out of Forward Bend, keep your spine supple and fluid. When you are standing, knees should be lifted and thighs engaged.

What if . . .

If doing the swan dive hurts your back, continue with the rolling up-and-down exercise instead.

Cool Thing

This is an *asana* you can work on anywhere.

Variation to Warm the Upper Body

- Circle the shoulders, keeping your movements fluid and relaxed. Repeat three or four times.
- Allowing the hand to lead, circle your arms, inhaling as arms come up, exhaling as arms go down. Repeat three or four times.
- Leading with the top of the head, roll down into Forward Bend with the knees bent, then reverse back up, keeping the movement slow and fluid.
- Folding at the hips, take a swan dive with straight legs into a Forward Bend on an exhale and reverse back up on an inhale.

TREE POSE (*Vrksasana*)

Mum

- Begin by standing in *tadasana* (Mountain Pose).
- Turn the left leg out to the side and bring your left foot to rest as high as it will go along the inside of the right leg. Give equal pressure from the right inner leg back into the foot. Resting the foot on the inside of your thigh is

the goal, but starting at the calf is perfectly acceptable. Avoid resting your foot against the inside of the knee, however.

- Straighten the standing leg and lift the kneecap to engage the leg muscles.
- Bring your palms together in front of your heart (unless you are holding your baby).
- Lengthen the spine and draw your navel in and up.
- Keep the hips level and the chest open. This is a good time to practice *mula bandha* (Kegel exercise).
- To increase the difficulty of this pose, extend your arms above your head, interlacing the fingers and pointing your index fingers to the ceiling.
- Imagine your upper body is weightless and the lower body is anchoring you to the ground.

Baby

If you are holding your baby in your arms, she can face in or out. If your baby is on the mat in front of your feet, imagine her resting in the shade of your "tree."

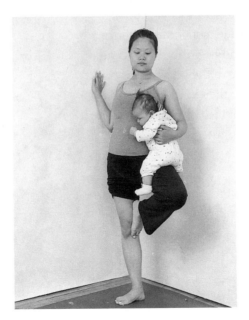

Tree Pose

Essentials

Keep the standing leg straight and the foot firmly planted on the mat.

What if . . .

If you feel unstable, move to a wall and use one hand for balance. Or allow your lifted foot to return to the mat for a moment and then back into the position.

Cool Thing

If you find your balance point you can feel completely weightless.

BABY ENGAGEMENT EXERCISE: LEOPARD SWING

This is a nice movement break before the standing poses continue. We call this the Leopard Swing because the babies remind us of leopard cubs hanging out on the branches of trees. Use one hand to support your baby's chest and head, and the other for her abdomen. Place your feet in a wide, comfortable stance, knees slightly bent, and begin to swing. Start with small swings close to the body and as you get more familiar with the exercise add variations including side to side (like a pendulum), forward and back, slow, fast, etc.

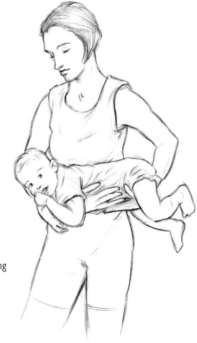

Leopard Swing

WARRIOR II (*Virabhadrasana II*)

Mum

- Place your feet in a wide stance, about .9 to 1.2 meters apart (approximately the length of your own leg).
- Keeping your hips facing forward, turn your right foot out to a 90-degree angle and the left foot in slightly.
- Line up the front heel in a straight line with the arch of the back foot.
- Press the outside edge and big toe joint of the back foot into the mat and keep your torso lifted as you bend your right knee to a right angle. The bent knee should be directly over the heel, and the weight should rest evenly along the bones of the foot.
- Lift your weight off your hips and lengthen your spine, keeping the back armpit over the back hip.
- Reach your back arm out to the side, parallel to the floor.
- Turn your head to face the bent leg and gaze forward.
- Hold for a few breaths to build stamina.
- Repeat on the other side.

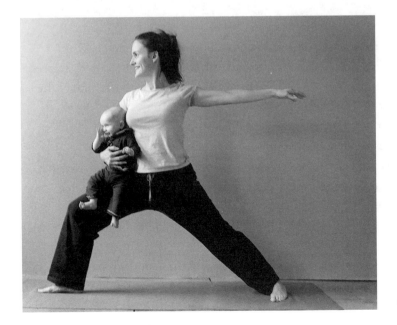

Warrior II

Baby

Your baby can sit and ride on your front thigh if her head control is good, or in your arms if she is too wobbly.

Essentials

Keep the length from head to tail.

What if . . .

If you feel pain in your front knee, decrease the 90-degree angle and make sure the outside of the bent knee is lined up with the pinkie toe.

Cool Thing

Imagine you are a warrior (it helps make the pose a little easier); feel the strength and power of the pose.

TRIANGLE POSE (*Trikonasana*)

Mum

- Place your feet in a wide stance, about .9 to 1.2 meters apart.
- With your hips facing forward, turn out your right foot 90 degrees and turn in the left foot slightly. The front heel lines up with the arch of the back foot.
- Extend your arms to the sides, parallel with the floor.
- Straighten the legs and lift the kneecaps.
- Lengthen and lift your waist.
- Reach your torso over the right leg by creasing at the right hip.
- Make sure the torso is extended in line with the front leg—not dipped in front.
- Place your right hand on the shin or ankle for support, and reach your left hand to the ceiling.
- Press the back heel down and extend through the top of the head.
- Open the front of your chest and allow your shoulder blades to slide down your back.

- Keep the abdominal muscles moving in as you take a few long breaths in this pose.
- Repeat on the other side.

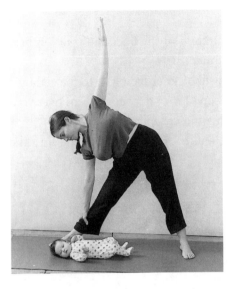
Triangle Pose

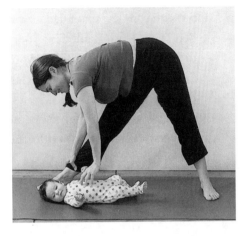
Triangle Variation

Baby
Your baby is lying by your front foot. When you change sides, turn around so that the other foot is next to your baby.

Essentials
Keep the sides of your waist reaching evenly. Imagine you are moving between two walls.

What if . . .
If you feel pressure or pain behind the front knee, work with it slightly bent.

Cool Thing
Triangle Pose is a fantastic stretch for the whole body, especially the hips and spine.

Variation to Entertain Your Baby
Circle the top arm over your head and past your baby, tickling him as you pass by. He will learn to anticipate each approaching arm circle.

HEAD TO KNEE POSE *(Janu Sirsasana)*

Mum

- Sit with your legs extended forward.
- Bend your left leg, allowing your knee to rest on the floor and your left heel to nestle against the inside of your left inner thigh.
- Press the back of the extended leg to the floor, knee facing up to the ceiling.
- Facing forward, with your chest wide, bend forward from the hips over your extended leg. Keep your spine long rather than rounded.
- Reach your hands forward to the calf, ankle, or foot, and breathe into the stretch.
- Repeat on the other side.

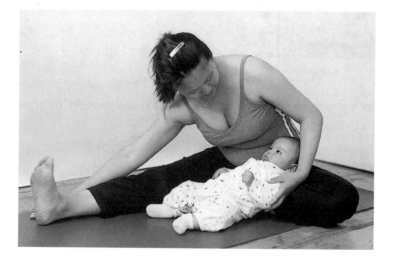

Head to Knee Pose

Baby

Your baby can nestle in the fold of your bent leg, or you can place your baby next to your extended leg facing you.

Essentials

Keep your weight evenly distributed to both sit bones and keep your torso extended as you fold forward.

What if . . .

If you can't place your heel on your upper thigh, work with it where it is comfortable.

Cool Thing

This pose combines a gentle twist with a Forward Bend so you are doing a lot all at once. It is said to tone the abdominal organs.

MODIFIED BOAT POSE (*Navasana*)

Mum

- Sit on the mat with your knees bent and feet on the floor.
- Hold your outer thighs and lift your chest.
- Keeping your abdominal muscles engaged and chest lifted, raise your feet just off the floor.
- Let your torso tilt back slightly for balance and keep your lower back moving up and in.
- If you can, raise your shins so that they are parallel to the floor and reach your hands toward your feet or, for added support, place your hands behind you on the floor.

Baby

Baby is on your lap facing you. If she is sitting securely, reach your hands toward your shins, palms facing your body.

Essentials

Your lower back and chest must be lifted.

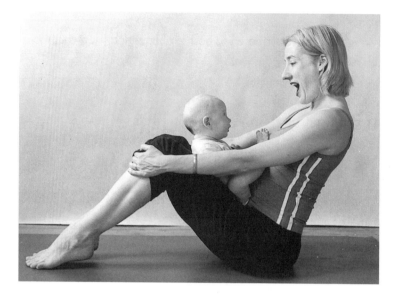

Modified Boat Pose

What if . . .

If you feel as though you are falling backward, move your feet farther away from your body or work with your feet on the floor until you build the strength you need to lift them without collapsing in the lower back.

Baby what if . . .

If your baby seems uncomfortable, she can face out, her belly on your thighs. This counts as tummy play, too!

Cool Thing

This pose takes considerable core strength, but it feels like less work because you're so close to your baby.

Variation to Stretch Back

- Start in Modified Boat Pose with your baby in your lap and your feet on the floor.
- Hold the sides of your thighs to lift your chest to face the ceiling.
- Round the spine, stretching away from your thighs (practice pulling your abdominal muscles in). Then sit up straight, lifting a little taller.
- Repeat three times.

LOCUST POSE (*Salabhasana*)

Mum

- Lie on your stomach, legs and feet extended behind you with the legs hip-width apart and parallel.
- Rest your hands along the sides of your torso with the knuckles on the floor.
- Inhale as you lift head, chest, and legs off the floor.
- Press your pubic bone into the mat and lengthen your lower back.
- Open your chest and allow your shoulder blades to slide down your back.
- Lift your torso as high as your feet.
- Keep your gaze on your baby and your head in line with your spine.
- Remain here for a few breaths and lower evenly back to the mat.

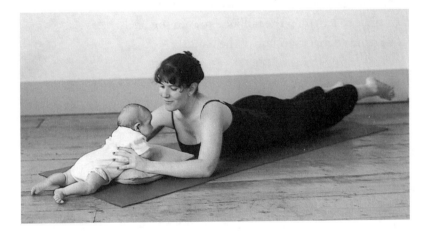

Locust Pose

Baby

Your baby is lying on her stomach, nose-to-nose with you. Tummy time!

Essentials

The pubic bone should press strongly into the mat and the legs should remain hip width apart and parallel.

What if . . .

If your legs move very far apart, lower them a little bit. If it is too much of a strain on your back to keep them raised, begin by allowing them to remain on the mat. Then work up to the full lift.

Cool Thing

Enjoy the novelty of being on your stomach, knowing that the pose tones your bladder and uterus and greatly strengthens the abdomen and lower back. Also, your baby will soon be able to join you in imitation of this pose.

Variation to Open Chest

- Interlace your fingers behind your back.
- As you lift your upper body, roll out your shoulders and reach your hands down toward your heels.
- Keep your gaze on your baby in front of you.
- Continue to lengthen the tailbone toward the heels.
- Lower and change the clasp of the hands.

BABY ENGAGEMENT EXERCISES: LOCUST TUMMY PLAY

In the Locust Pose, both mother and baby are on their stomachs (see page 65). If your baby is younger than eight weeks you may want to prop her up on a cushion, which will slightly elevate her torso. Locust may feel strange to you as well, after so many months of protecting your abdomen and lying on your back or sides. Nevertheless, these poses present a great opportunity to model a position for your baby that strengthens everyone's back muscles.

Mum

Sit cross-legged and do these simple baby exercises.

Baby

Your baby is lying on her belly in front of you.

BABY'S ARMS

- Try to uncurl your baby's fingers and place each palm on the floor near her shoulders (see page 28).
- Use finger openers like rubbing the knuckles together, or stroking palms (see page 27).
- Gently fold one of your baby's feet in toward the opposite buttock, then extend her leg. Repeat on the other side.

MASSAGE

- Give a general massage, stroking from your baby's neck to her buttocks, hand over hand.
- Using one finger, gently stroke the length of her spine from the back of her neck to her tailbone. (This encourages a back arch and head lift.) Also, using your fingertips, stroke from the spine out, around the rib cage, toward the front ribs.
- Give little squeezes down the backs of baby's legs followed by long strokes.
- Massage soles of her feet, out through each toe in turn.

SOLES OF THE FEET TOGETHER

With your baby lying on his stomach, pat and rub the soles of his feet together (see page 29).

FROGGY

With your baby on his stomach, place your hands against the soles of his feet (like a little wall). Keep your hands very stable. Baby will push against your hands and straighten his knees. This is an instinctive action and a preparation for crawling.

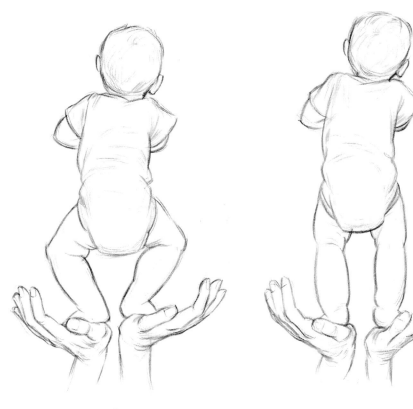

Froggy I (bent legs)   Froggy II (straight legs)

HALF WHEEL POSE *(Setu Bandhasana)*

Mum

- Lie on your back with your knees bent and your feet on the floor close to the sit bones.
- Inhale, and on the exhale draw the navel strongly toward the floor, engaging your abdominal muscles.
- Press your feet into the mat to lift the hips and roll up and down along the spine slowly, repeating the movement a few times.
- Keep your knees parallel and press the big toe joints into the mat.
- Keep your collarbones broad and draw the shoulder blades together underneath you.
- On the last roll, stay up for several breaths and feel the backs of your legs and gluteal muscles working.

Baby

- Position your baby on your chest or upper abdomen either lying down or in a semi-seated position, supported by your thighs. She will ride up and down as you move through the pose.
- Exhale and move your head up gently toward your baby and make eye contact with her each time you lift up.
- Kiss your baby as you work your upper abdominals.

Essentials

Hollow your abdominal muscles and lengthen your tailbone so that you roll sequentially through the spine. There will be a slight natural curve as you rest in a neutral position. When in the resting position, make sure to keep your sacrum on the floor.

What if . . .

If you feel a strain in your lower back, press your feet into the mat to help lengthen your back, and lift your spine only a few centimeters off the floor. Don't practice the variations until you are more comfortable in this pose.

Cool Thing

Besides strengthening the core of the body, this *asana* massages your back as you roll up and down the spine.

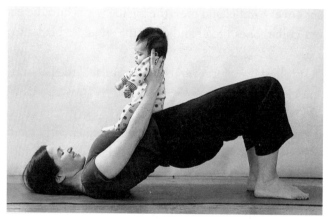

Half Wheel Pose
(hips up)

Variation 1

- With your back flat on the floor, exhale, drawing the navel to the spine.
- Lift your head and look at your baby leaning against thighs or on your lap. (Keep the navel drawn in!)
- Relax head to the floor. Repeat 5 to 10 times.

Variation 2 (*Without Your Baby*)

- Bend your knees into your chest, and slowly lower them to the mat.
- Keep your back long, navel moving to the spine. Repeat five times.

BABY ENGAGEMENT IN HALF WHEEL

These exercises are the most basic in our Flying Child Pose series. They are designed for babies six weeks and older; before that your baby should rest on your chest. This series adds abdominal work to your practice and offers a whole new vantage point from which your baby can watch you. Babies love this active form of play; it is fun for all involved. Feel free to add variations as you see fit.

Flying Child Pose I

Mum

- Begin by lying on your back with your knees bent and your feet on the floor.
- Fold your knees into your chest.

Baby

- Your baby is lying tummy down on your shins.
- Wrap your hands around her sides with your fingers spread wide, spanning her ribs.
- Gently bounce your baby by bouncing your shins at a slow pace.

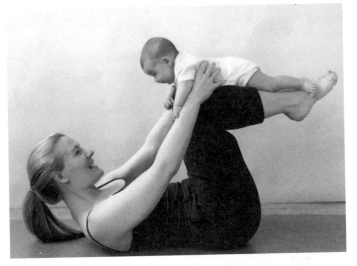

Flying Child Pose I

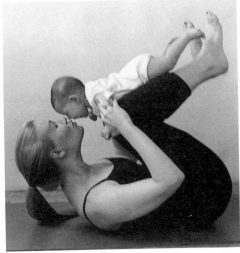

Flying Child Pose (with a kiss)

- Gradually increase size and speed of bounces, letting your baby's enjoyment and security guide you.
- Gently rock your knees from side to side (not too far in either direction).
- Extend your shins slightly away from you and bring them back in. (This will engage your lower abdominals.) Make sure your shins stay parallel to the floor. Gradually increase repetitions.
- Lift your head and bring your knees (and her face) to your nose for a kiss.

SAGE POSE *(Bharadvajasana I)*

Mum
- Start by sitting on your heels.
- Shift your hips to the left until the left hip rests on the mat.
- Use your right hand against the left thigh to rotate your torso to the left, placing the left hand on the floor behind you.
- Keep the right hip moving down away from your waist and lift your chest up and around to the left.
- Broaden the collarbones.

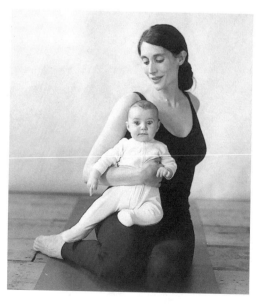

Sage Pose

- Think of twisting around a central axis.
- Hold for three to five breaths.

Baby
- Your baby is sitting on your lap, supported by your right arm as you twist to the left.
- Turn your head to gaze back at him, releasing your tight neck muscles. Use your hand to keep him safely on your lap.

Essentials
Keep the back hip descending toward the mat and your spine long.

What if . . .
If you feel discomfort in the lower back, relax the twist in the hips and work on the rotation in the upper body.

Cool Thing
This is a great release for the spine without being too strong a twist. Also, you can do it while nursing.

SEATED FORWARD BEND (*Paschimottanasana*)

Mum
- Sit with both legs extended and your knees and toes pointing to the ceiling.
- Lift from your waist and press the backs of the legs into the floor.
- Keep your collarbones wide and shoulder blades dropped down.
- Bend forward from the hips, and keep your torso as long as possible over straight legs. Think about reaching your lower ribs to knees, sternum toward feet.
- Keep your legs extended and the lower back broad.
- Your arm can rest lightly on your baby or reach for the outsides of your feet.

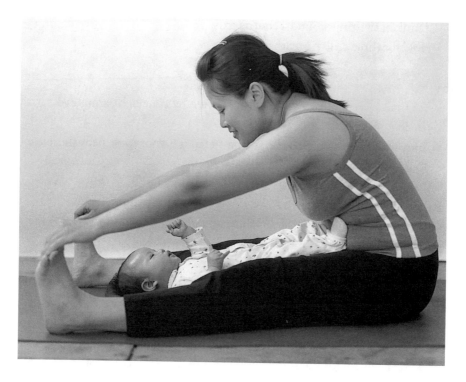

Seated Forward Bend

Baby

- Place your baby on her back, cradled between your legs.
- As you bend forward, make eye contact and if you can reach her (with a straight spine) give her a kiss.

Essentials

Move forward on an exhale, evenly and with no bouncing.

What if . . .

If your back hurts, or you have difficulty bending forward, sit on a pillow to lift the lower back, or let your knees bend slightly.

Cool Thing

Your baby will entice you forward, taking your mind off the intensity of the stretch.

RESTING POSE *(Savasana)*

Mum

- Lie on your back with your hips a few centimeters from the chair.
- Place your calves on the seat of the chair.
- Relax your whole body, especially your lower abdomen.
- Rest here for five minutes or longer.

Baby

Your baby can lie on your chest or abdomen, tummy down, or she can rest beside you in her own *savasana*.

Essentials

Be present with your breath and with your baby.

What if . . .

If your legs feel as if they need to roll out, let them. If you get cold, cover yourself with a blanket.

Cool Thing

This pose relieves back tension you may have experienced. It is very relaxing mentally and physically. Imagine that time spent in this pose is time spent letting the body heal.

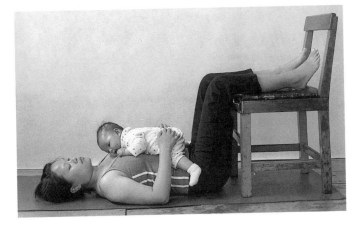

Resting Pose
(legs on chair)

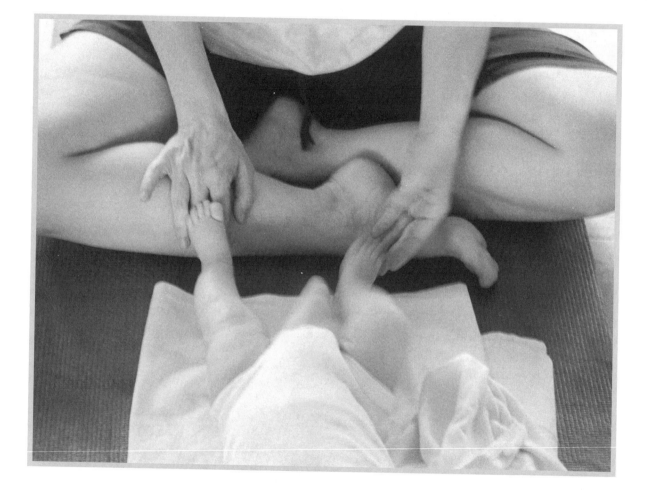

5

CLASS 2:
Three to Six Months

A CLASS FOR ENERGIZING AND OPENING
APPROXIMATELY 45 MINUTES; HOLD EACH POSE FOR FIVE BREATHS.

Breathing Exercise: Alternate Nostril Breathing

Seated Twist

Wide-Leg Stretch and Side Bend Variation

Sun Salute, Series II

Awkward Pose and Twist Variation

Warrior 1

Flank Pose

Wide-Leg Forward Bend and Twist Variation

Seated Spinal Twist

Head to Knee Pose

Locust Pose with Leg Variation

Full Bow

Camel Pose

Half Wheel Pose and Variations

Lying-Down Twist

Resting Pose with Supported Knees

Our second class focuses on your baby's third to sixth months. Physically and psychologically, this is often a time when new mothers experience the feeling that their lives are beginning to return to normal. Not completely, but getting there. Your baby is no longer considered a newborn and is probably developing a more consistent routine of sleeping, eating, bathing, and other waking activities. This slight increase in her independence allows you to actually plan your time. The task of boiling an egg will no longer seem as daunting as constructing a seven-course meal. The baby is still calling many of the shots, however, and you will still feel as if you're being pulled in several different directions at once. Frustration and the early glimmerings of normalcy coexist like new friends from different parts of the world.

Although you may still feel tired and somewhat overwhelmed by the responsibility of caring for a baby, you are probably getting more sleep. Sleep deprivation can be a major cause of depression, and it's amazing how your brain begins to function better on just a little more rest. We remember a friend with a newborn calling us in tears after an untold number of sleepless nights. She felt she was a terrible mother, and that every one of her daughter's complaints was due to her own personal failings. When her baby was three months of age, she started getting a little consistent sleep and experienced less chronic fragility. Suddenly, because both she and her baby were sleeping better, her mood turned a corner. At times we lose sight of the powerful healing effects of sleep. Getting an afternoon "power nap" or an extra hour at night can go a long way toward improving your worldview.

After three months together, you know your baby better. You are accustomed to the nuances of his cries and little personal habits. You delight in his emerging personality. You have been an integral part of his growth up to this point and have witnessed many changes. While this is thrilling, you may also experience an odd sense of loss as each developmental milestone is passed and wax nostalgic about the first few months of your baby's life. Although you may sometimes feel overcome by the sheer magnitude of your baby's physical needs—the constant diaper changes, feedings, spitting up, bathing, drooling, and so on—there is also something comforting in the immediacy and intimacy of satisfying these needs.

You may also have expected that things (like your body, for instance) would have been restored to normalcy more quickly, and you are now realizing that this is not the case. We have often felt the need to remind others (and ourselves) that three months is not a long time, and we all need to exercise patience as much as possible.

We also may have people around us (including our loved ones) who counted on us to snap back to exactly the person we used to be, like some postpartum Barbie doll. People may expect you to have "recovered." You've had your time off (as if you'd had some kind of vacation) and now you are supposed to bounce back to business as usual, whether or not you're returning to work. Instead, you feel like Rip Van Winkle emerging into an utterly foreign world. Indeed, maternity leaves of perhaps a few weeks, intended to be generous, pressure us to return to work. But even women eager to return to the job feel anxious when they leave their baby behind to return to the workplace. Saying good-bye at the door to an infant can be extremely stressful. It's often the mothers who go through separation anxiety. Give yourself time to sort out all the demands being made on you. If you do return to work, these Baby Om classes can provide a nourishing haven in which you can reconnect with your infant while shrugging off the stresses of the workday.

The Class

The *asanas* in this section all share the qualities of strengthening the body from the core out and opening the chest to increase energy. The arching in the standing poses encourages the body to become receptive to the more intense chest opening and back bending. Back bending can be challenging for the lower back, so you must work slowly and mindfully. If low back pain occurs during or after the practice, do less and alternate this class with Class 1. The side bend creates length in the spine, and the twisting releases the back. Practicing these poses will build heat in the body and will work to relieve daily tensions. All of these poses improve posture and alignment. It is important to build stamina and strength, so holding each pose for the recommended duration is an important goal. Despite all the focus on stamina in this class it is important to listen to your own body and follow its cues. Adjust your efforts and your expectations in accordance with how you feel on each day.

The more awareness you bring to your breath—keeping it smooth and even—the warmer your body becomes and the deeper the effects of the *asanas*. This is a good time to push your body a little more. You're ready for it. You'll find it amazing how quietly exhilarating this can be.

Your Body

At this point, you are still carrying around a very young baby for much of the day. The most common baby-holding posture is with your hips jutting forward, using your hips as both support and brakes. This stance compresses your lower back while rounding your upper back. It puts a great deal of strain on the lower back and increases the tightness in the hips, which further strains the lower back, shoulders, and neck. We felt as if we went from healthy alignment to imitating the snake man at Coney Island within a matter of months, and would shriek when we caught a glimpse of our profile in a mirror. How did this happen so quickly? With this posture, low back pain is no stranger, and it is one of the most common complaints we hear. It's a difficult habit to break, and if your breasts are heavy due to nursing, the problem is exacerbated.

This is the time for you to become aware of the relationship between how you hold your baby and your posture. Notice how you sit and stand when nursing or feeding, doing chores, walking with your baby, even brushing your teeth. These *asanas* will help you to find a more lifted and open vertical alignment, which is essential for protecting your lower back.

Other less dire things you may be experiencing during this time are hair loss (Sarah's personal favorite), dehydration (Laura's), and a general run-down feeling. Your abdomen will still be soft and you will want to spend this period working with your abdominal muscles, pelvic floor, and torso alignment. If you suspect that your central abdominal muscles have separated during pregnancy (a common condition known as *diastasis*), you need to work especially carefully during back bends. Recovery from this condition requires a slower approach to any pose that stretches your abdomen. (See chapter 11 on postpartum conditions.)

Although abdominal work is essential, don't make the mistake of overworking the stomach by doing excessive repetitions. Less is more with abdominal work. Kegels are an essential part of abdominal work, since the pelvic floor supports the abdominal cavity. Doing simple exercises like the Boat Pose, Awkward Pose, or Half Wheel, with the navel drawn in toward the spine and the pelvic floor lifted in a Kegel, will tone those muscles better than doing a hundred crunches. We encourage you to work both the front and back of your body equally for alignment and flexibility. Sit-ups themselves don't eliminate fat, and if done incorrectly, tighten the front of the body and aggravate already tight shoulders and neck. Remember that for now, rebuilding strength is far more important than losing extra kilos. In addition, learning how to release excess abdominal tension (as in forward bending) is an art unto itself and immensely important for deepening the poses.

The opening poses in this series also help to release the diaphragm (breathing muscle) and extend the deep abdominal muscles as well as the front of the chest. By opening the chest you start to work the muscles of the upper back, and the stronger your back and arms become, the less you will strain your neck and shoulders. If it sounds as if we are repeating ourselves, it's only because we've experienced this so dramatically. An ex-dancer and mother of two recently told us she hasn't stood up straight in five years. We believe her!

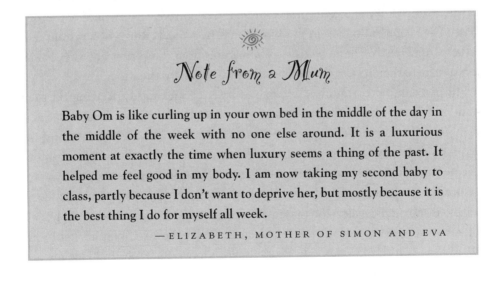

Note from a Mum

Baby Om is like curling up in your own bed in the middle of the day in the middle of the week with no one else around. It is a luxurious moment at exactly the time when luxury seems a thing of the past. It helped me feel good in my body. I am now taking my second baby to class, partly because I don't want to deprive her, but mostly because it is the best thing I do for myself all week.

—ELIZABETH, MOTHER OF SIMON AND EVA

Your Baby

During this period, babies begin to work on more complex coordinated movements. They gain upper-body strength and control, and may roll over. They can sit up with assistance and will often try to do so on their own as they reach for interesting objects. Accomplishments such as grasping toys and letting them go, putting their hands in their mouths, and initiating and breaking gaze are important aspects of their play and development. Their movements have become smoother and less jerky. As they move, kicking their legs and swinging their arms, their hands may come into view and become their most fascinating new toys. As they begin to handle objects, they are replacing reflexive movements with deliberate ones and starting to understand that they have some degree of control in their world. This is a critical aspect of their developing sense of identity. Coupled with the honing of hand-eye coordination these months might be known as the "everything in mouth" period.

Most babies are learning to hold their heads up and can support their own head if gently lifted from a prone to a sitting position. As soon as they do this, they become more involved in the world around them. A baby's muscular control occurs in two directions. If you imagine a wave from top to bottom, that is, head to toe, one phase of development travels in this direction. The second "wave" occurs from central to peripheral. As the nervous system matures from the center outward, babies gain control of their torsos, then limbs, fingers, and finally, their toes.

In preparation for rolling over, babies practice kicking while lying on their backs, and lifting their heads and shoulders while lying on their tummies. Some begin to sit up, an essential step in the development of strength in the lumbar spine for postural support in standing and walking. Sitting also allows your baby to become part of the social scene, something that is becoming increasingly important to him. The exercises in this class will give your baby an opportunity to practice all of these things and develop the muscular awareness necessary for the next physical milestones. To prepare for crawling (in what seems like the distant future, but comes sooner than you think) your baby must learn to move his limbs individually and then to coordinate them. The series of exercises in which each limb is moved independently, combined with the opposing arm and leg movement exercises, addresses these important coordinations. Time spent lying on the belly helps build the necessary arm and torso strength. The rolling exercise teaches your baby a method of locomotion, giving him a way to change his vantage point and gain independence.

Although colic may be receding, this can still be a fussy period. Babies may begin cutting teeth at this time, which may put them out of sorts. New experiences can help to distract them from their discomfort whether it's due to colic or teething, so try some different moves and surprise them. Add a tummy tickle as you bend forward; lift her over your head as you go from Forward Bend to standing. Sarah was able to really enjoy her daughter Rosey (who was often colicky) during this interactive play. The *asanas* provided moments where they could have fun and bond in a way that was difficult to achieve in other circumstances. The swinging series includes several different planes of movement: up and down, around, forward and back. Most babies love this because it stimulates their vestibular system, the system that allows you to keep your balance, maintain an upright position, and accomplish fluid movement.

By three months your baby is forming strong interpersonal connections. He is chortling and laughing with you, smiling and reaching for your face, grabbing your hair, and beginning to master the skills and strength necessary for interacting with other people. Babies progress rapidly and will absorb about as much as you can provide.

Be a gentle aid in your baby's practice. Help him attain a skill or put him through a new motion.

ALTERNATE NOSTRIL BREATHING

The breathing exercise we recommend for the period of 3–6 months is called Alternate Nostril Breathing. The description may sound a little daunting, but stay with it. It can be deeply balancing and calming, and we love it.

- Sit in a chair or on the mat (with a pillow under your hips).
- Take a few inhalations and exhalations of even length to prepare.
- Fold the pointer and middle finger of your right hand into your palm, leaving your thumb, fourth finger, and pinky extended.
- Lightly touch the fourth finger and thumb together and then release.
- Take the hand to the bridge of your nose, with the tip of the thumb on the right side and tip of the fourth finger on the left.
- Inhale a breath, then, as you exhale gently, block the left nostril with your fourth finger and breathe out through the right nostril.
- Inhale through the right nostril, then block the right side with the thumb and exhale through the left.
- Inhale through the left, then block the left side and exhale right.
- Make each inhale and exhale last the same amount of time. It may help to start with three slow counts for each inhale and exhale. You can experiment with different counts to find your natural timing.
- Repeat for 5–10 cycles (right and left is one cycle). End on an exhale through the right nostril.
- When this feels comfortable, you can also add a slight breath retention (hold) at the end of each inhalation.

SEATED TWIST (Parsva Siddhasana)

Mum

- Sit cross-legged on the mat, pressing down with the sit bones while lengthening the spine and head toward the ceiling.
- Broaden across the collarbones and imagine lifting your heart.
- Place your left hand on the outside of your right knee, and your right hand on the floor behind you.
- Keep lifted as you rotate your rib cage around to the right. To support and

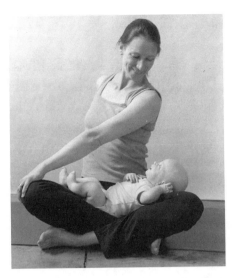

Seated Twist

deepen the twist, use a slight pressure of the left hand into the right knee as the back hand presses into the mat.

- Keep your chest wide and waist lifted as you deepen the twist gently with each exhale.
- Relax your neck as you enjoy your twist.
- Repeat on the other side.
- Return to the center, sit still, and chant *Om* to your baby.
- After you have finished your *Om*(s), practice your Kegels.

Baby

Rest your baby in your lap, sitting or reclining. Smile and gaze at her as you experiment with changing your focus. Play peek-a-boo!

Essentials
Keep the weight even in both sit bones.

What if . . .
If you can't reach your back hand to the mat, move it closer to your body or place your hand on a book.

Cool Thing
You can keep on twisting and twisting.

Variation for Seated Twist

- Sit in a cross-legged position.
- Rotate to the right using your hands as in Seated Twist.
- Bend to the side, bringing your left shoulder to the left knee.
- Keep the right shoulder and arm extended to the ceiling.
- Look at your baby.
- Repeat on the other side.

WIDE-LEG STRETCH (*Upavistha Konasana*)

Mum

- Open your legs in a wide V with the legs straight and the knees and toes pointing toward the ceiling.
- Bring your arms forward, fingertips lightly touching the mat in front of you.
- Lift the spine and widen the front of the body.
- Descend your weight into the sit bones and keep them pressing into the mat.
- Extend your torso forward, walking your hands ahead of you on either side of your baby.
- Keep the front, back, and sides of the body long.

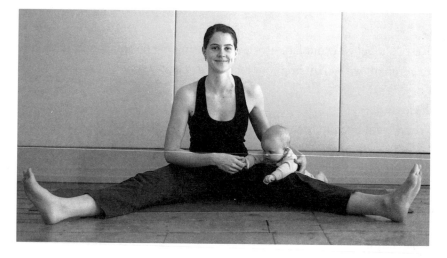

Wide-Leg Stretch

Baby

Your baby may be placed on the mat between your legs and you can bend forward over her, or she can lean across one thigh as you extend your torso forward. In this position, she will help you keep your leg flat on the floor while she gains strength in her back and neck extensors. In the side bend variation, if you lay your baby on the inside of the leg you will be bending over, you can tickle and coo as you move toward her.

Essentials

In the side bend variation, the opposing hip must stay on the floor. Don't let your hip pop up.

What if . . .

If your back rounds in this pose, try sitting on a pillow to lift your hips slightly.

Cool Thing

This *asana* is a universal warm-up—it always works.

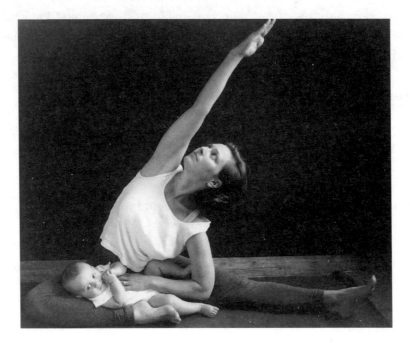

Side Bend Variation

Side Bend Variation
- Press the right hip down as you stretch over your left leg.
- Rest your left arm near the left shin or ankle.
- Keep your chest facing front and the side ribs facing the ceiling.
- Keep both sides of torso very long.
- Extend the top arm overhead toward the left foot.
- Move both shoulders down and away from your ears.
- Repeat on the other side.
- If lower back and torso are particularly tight, bend the opposing leg in.

BABY ENGAGEMENT IN WIDE-LEG STRETCH

Now that your baby is stronger and more acclimated to his environment, he loves basking in your attention. He will begin to practice rolling over and sitting up, two thrilling achievements. These exercises help him gain awareness of his arms and legs and develop deep abdominal support. Either sit with your legs wide, stretching your hamstrings, or sit in a comfortable cross-legged position while you work your baby's legs, hips, arms, and torso individually and in cross-patterning (left with right, right with left).

For Your Baby's Legs

Mum
Sit with legs in a V or cross-legged.

Baby
Your baby is lying on his back with his feet toward you.

Leg Extensions
- Holding your baby's calves, gently bend both his knees in toward his chest three to six times.
- Bicycle one knee at a time in toward his chest. Repeat eight times on each leg.
- Holding your baby's ankles, roll his feet up toward his forehead and back down again. Repeat two to four times.

- Bring one knee at a time diagonally across his chest. Repeat two to four times.

Leg Rotations
- Hold your baby's shins and bring his knees to his chest.
- Gently open his knees wide, and then bring them back together before straightening his legs. Repeat from the beginning four times.
- Place one hand lightly on your baby's hip to keep that hip from rocking as you lift the opposite leg. Repeat three times on each leg.
- Keeping one hand on his hip, make little leg circles in both directions with the lifted leg. Make three circles with each leg in each direction.
- Gently rotate his ankles in little circles. Do this in both directions on both sides.

Massage
- Give little squeezes down each leg.
- Follow this with long extending strokes down each leg.
- Stroke the soles of his feet and wiggle each toe.

For Your Baby's Arms

Arm extensions
- Hold your baby's hands and gently open his arms wide to the side and close them across his chest. Make sure to alternate which arm is on top.
- Lift his arms high over his head then down toward his waist. Repeat three to five times.
- Circle his arms in both directions three times.
- Move one arm up overhead and the other down. Repeat two to four times for each side.

Massage
- Squeeze lightly down your baby's arms.
- Give long strokes from his chest to his fingertips.
- Stroke the palm of each hand and massage to the end of each finger.

For Your Baby's Torso

Opposite arm and leg

This exercise helps the baby coordinate the right and left sides of her body in preparation for crawling.

- Hold the ankle and wrist of opposite arm and leg (for example, the right arm and left leg).
- Bring her hand and foot to touch at midpoint over her chest.
- Extend the hand and foot out, away from each other on the diagonal.
- Repeat four times on each side.

Rolling

Sit in a comfortable position on the floor with your baby on his back and facing you. Hold your baby's right calf and gently bring it across his left leg as in a twist three times, each one successively bigger. On the third cross help your baby roll all the way over onto his stomach. If his left arm gets caught, just lift the left hip to free it. Supporting his head, return him to his back and repeat with the other side.

Sitting

Gently hold your baby's hands and wrists and lead him up to a sitting position. Make sure his head is not dropping backward; if it is, support the back of his neck

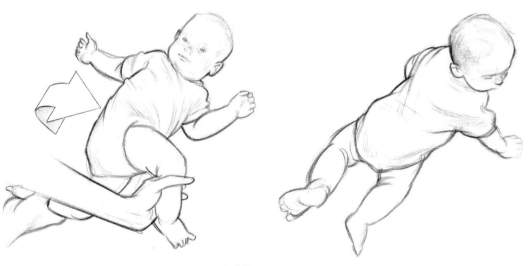

Roll (I)   Roll (II)

with your hands. Babies will often try to stand by pushing against the floor with their feet. If your baby initiates this, follow his lead and help him push up to standing, supporting his weight. Notice how pleased he is with himself! Gently sit him back down. Holding his arms to support his weight, roll him back through his spine to a reclining position (only from the seated position). Repeat from sitting to reclining two to four times.

To Finish

Sit in a cross-legged position and hug your baby to your chest. Circle your torso in medium-sized circles in both directions. Bring your torso to center and, if your baby is light enough, raise her over your head, lifting from your back and arms (not shoulders), and then bend your arms to bring her back to your chest for a kiss. Lift and lower two to four times.

SUN SALUTE, SERIES II (Surya Namaskar)

Baby lies on Mum's mat throughout this linked series of poses.

Mountain Pose (Tadasana)

- Stand with feet baby-width apart.
- Inhale, your arms overhead, palms together.

Forward Bend (Uttanasana)

- Exhale and swan dive forward over straight legs, keeping an extended spine.
- Keep the front of your body very long and your abdomen relaxed.

Lunge

- Inhale in Forward Bend and step your right leg straight behind you, placing the knee on the floor. Your front leg is bent so that the knee falls directly over the ankle.
- Exhale and stretch the front of your thigh, easing the pelvis toward the floor.

Downward Facing Dog (Adho Mukha Svanasana)

- Inhale in Lunge and step your left foot into Downward Facing Dog. Exhale.

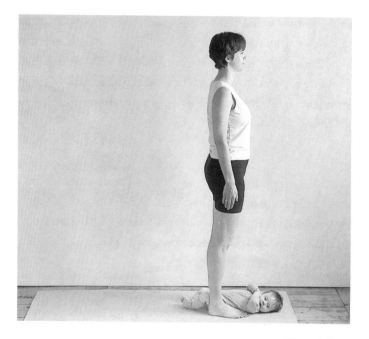

Mountain Pose

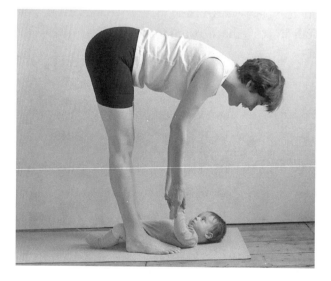

Forward Bend

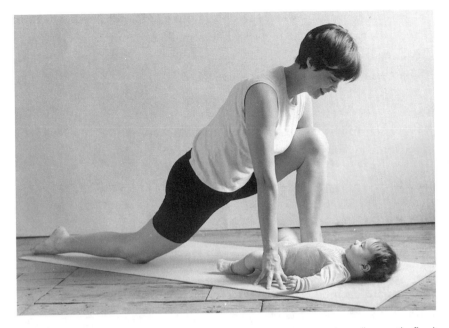

Lunge (knee on the floor)

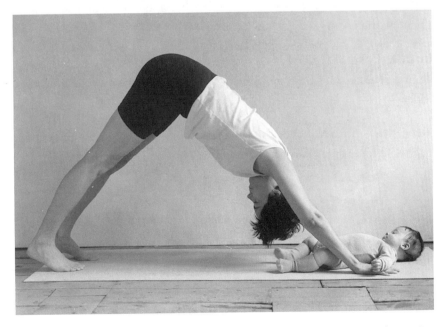

Downward Facing Dog

- Your feet are slightly wider than hip-width apart; your pelvis is floating up and back toward the ceiling; your knees are lifted; and your heels are moving back and down.
- Draw your navel in toward the spine.

Plank

- From Downward Facing Dog pose, inhale, chest and head forward so that you form one long, extended line from head to heel.

To Finish

Downward Facing Dog (*Adho Mukha Svanasana*)
Exhale back into Downward Facing Dog.

Lunge
From Downward Facing Dog, inhale and move your right leg next to your right hand. Your left knee is on the floor.

Forward Bend (*Uttanasana*)
Inhale and step the left leg forward to the left hand, moving you back into a Forward Bend. Exhale.

Mountain Pose (*Tadasana*)
Inhale and reverse swan-dive up into Mountain Pose. Exhale your arms down to your sides.

Repeat the entire sequence. Make two to four complete cycles. You can move through them more quickly as you warm up.

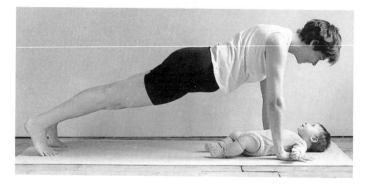

Plank

AWKWARD POSE *(Utkatasana)*

Mum

- Stand in *tadasana*, feet hip-width apart.
- On an inhale, slowly bend your knees and fold at the hips as if you were about to sit in a chair.
- Draw your navel in toward the spine, and keeping your weight moving down into your heels, apply *mula bandha* (pelvic floor lift).
- Breathe evenly in this position—this is a difficult *asana*.
- If you are holding your baby, move her into the hip crease as you sit, close to your center. If not, your arms can extend overhead, shoulder-width apart, continuing the line of the torso.
- Reach the top of the head and tips of the ears away from the tailbone to avoid swayback.

Baby

Your baby can sit in your lap facing outward or she can lie on the floor between your feet.

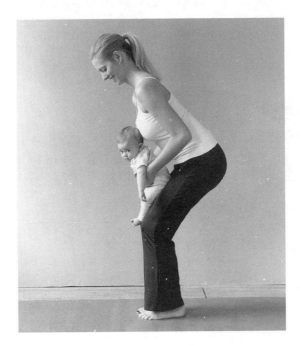

Awkward Pose

Essentials
Keep your legs parallel.

What if . . .
If your lower back hurts, you may be arching too much, or not engaging your lower abdominals. Keep the navel drawn into the spine, release the front of the hips, and lengthen sacrum down.

Cool Thing
This pose really heats you up.

TWIST VARIATION OF AWKWARD POSE *(Utkatasana)*

If the standard *asana* feels manageable, try this variation.

- While in *utkatasana*, place your palms together in front of your heart.
- Maintain the bend in the knees and good abdominal engagement.

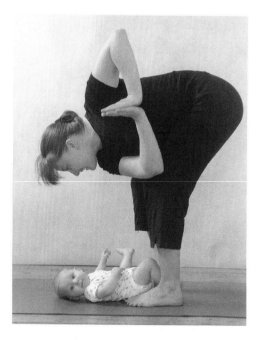

Awkward Pose
Twist Variation

- Spiral your rib cage around to the left, bend forward, and brace your right elbow on the outside of your left knee.
- Breathe into the twist and spiral rib cage around even further.
- Make sure your knees stay parallel.
- Gaze at your baby.
- Repeat on the other side.

BABY ENGAGEMENT EXERCISE: CIRCLES

- Hold your baby facing in or out, move your legs into a wide stance, and sway side to side taking a dip between each sway (think of a pendulum). Continue as long as you feel comfortable.
- Let the sway culminate in a full circle to the right. Turn in place and repeat three times stopping between each rotation. Repeat on the left side.
- Do this in front of a mirror for added fun. Be sure to allow enough time between each rotation for your baby's eyes to refocus.

WARRIOR I (Virabhadrasana I)

Mum
- Stand with your legs about 1.2 meters apart.
- Turn the right foot out 90 degrees and the left foot in 45 degrees.
- Turn your hips and torso to face the right foot.
- Bend the right knee, attempting to get the right thigh parallel to the floor. Do not allow your knee to move ahead of the ankle. If you need to, take a wider stance.
- Keep the back leg straight and the back heel reaching into the floor.
- Draw the pubic bone toward the navel for support, and reach long through the spine.
- Widen across your chest and keep your heart high.
- If you are not holding your baby, your arms should reach forward and up toward the ceiling.

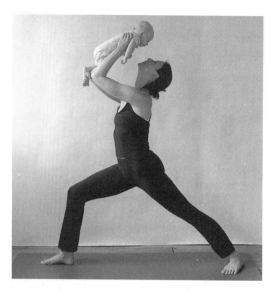

Warrior I

Baby

Your baby can sit on your front thigh, facing out. She can practice head control and sitting up as you spiral your torso toward her. Try to lift her overhead and bend your elbows as you bring her in for kisses.

Essentials

Try to keep your back heel down. Narrow your stance if it won't stay down.

What if . . .

If you feel compression in the lower back you are probably throwing your shoulders back too far. Keep the shoulders over the hips and remember to engage the lower abdomen and lift in the front of the body.

Cool Thing

It is virtually impossible to get both hips facing front, and you may spend a lifetime of practice trying.

Arm Variation

If you are not holding your baby, try clasping your hands behind your head, reaching your elbows wide to each side. This stretches the pectorals and deepens the curve of the upper back.

FLANK POSE *(Parsvottanasana)*

Mum

- Stand with legs about .9 to 1.2 meters apart.
- Turn the right foot out 90 degrees and turn the left foot in until the legs are almost parallel (the back foot will remain slightly turned out).
- Turn your hips and torso to face the right foot.
- Bring your hands to your hips, pulling your shoulders long, away from your neck.
- Press the back heel down, lifting and opening the chest.
- Begin to fold forward from the hips over the right thigh, keeping the chest opened and both sides of the torso extended.
- Stop at a point halfway into your Forward Bend to extend the spine even longer and square your hips again. Try to keep your right hip from shifting forward and out to the side.
- Release into your deepest Forward Bend, sternum reaching toward the ankle, and hands to the floor.
- The weight should feel evenly distributed between the front and back foot.
- Smile and blow kisses at your baby.
- Repeat on the other side.

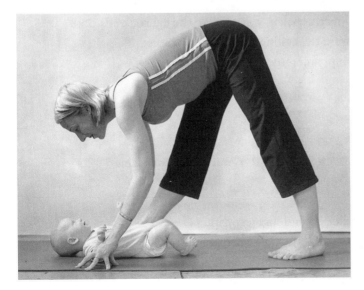

Flank Pose Forward Bend

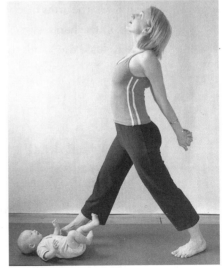

Chest Opening Variation

Baby

Your baby is on the mat next to your front foot. As you bend forward you can grab hold of her hands and do some arm wiggles. Your baby can practice sitting up, leaning against your leg as you support her weight with your hands.

Essentials

Keep your hips square facing over the front leg.

What if . . .

If your hamstrings feel too tight to allow much forward bend, hold as far forward as you can with a flat back until your hamstring stretch increases.

Cool Thing

You really feel the stretch in the front leg hamstring.

Chest Opening Variation

- Interlace the fingers behind the lower back.
- Stretch the arms straight, palms together, and lift the chest.
- If you can't get your hands together, hold your wrists or elbows behind your back and lift the chest.
- Keep the arms reaching directly back as you come to the flat back position.
- Lift the hands slightly toward the ceiling—open a little more.
- Release the hands to the hips and return to upright.

WIDE-LEG FORWARD BEND (Prasarita Padottanasana)

Mum

- Stand with your feet parallel, about four feet apart.
- Stand tall, lifting the torso out of the hips without arching.
- Lift the kneecaps and roll the inner thigh back.
- Bend forward to the mat, keeping the spine long.
- Place your fingertips on the ground on either side of your baby.

- Draw the navel toward the spine.
- Send your sit bones up and your heels down, keeping the hips directly over the heels.
- Broaden across the lower back as you release forward with your head toward your baby.

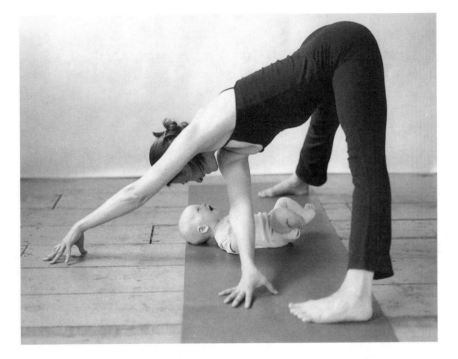

Wide-Leg Forward Bend (Variation Spine Stretch)

Baby

Your baby is on the mat between your legs, or slightly in front of you. Cuddle with her and make eye contact as you bend forward.

Essentials

Keep the legs straight; kneecaps and the arch of the foot lifted.

What if . . .

If you can't reach the ground, widen your legs or place your hands on a chair or wall.

Cool Thing

In this pose you can get a lot done all at once. It delivers a great stretch for the hips and back, tones the abdomen, and calms the mind and quiets the nervous system. It also has great peek-a-boo potential.

Variation Spine Stretch

- From the forward bending position, lift your back parallel to the floor with a long spine.
- Walk your hands forward, keeping your hips over your heels.
- Stretch fully from fingertips to sit bones.
- Return to your Forward Bend. Add a twist by reaching the right arm underneath the left arm and walk fingers toward the left foot.

SEATED SPINAL TWIST *(Marichyasana III)*

Mum

- Sit with your legs extended in front of you.
- Bend your right knee toward the ceiling and place the right foot on the floor with the right ankle touching the inner-left thigh.
- Sit upright. Lift the chest using your hands on the bent knee for support.
- Begin to rotate toward the bent knee, keeping the spine long.
- Hook your left elbow or hand around the right knee.
- Inhale, and on an exhale deepen the twist to the right.
- Keep your collarbones wide, your waist long, the top of your head moving toward the ceiling, and the shoulders down and away from your ears.
- Repeat on the other side.

Baby

Your baby is sitting on your extended leg, facing forward or out over the left arm. If he is sitting up, you can support him with your working arm, holding on to the back of your thigh instead of your knee.

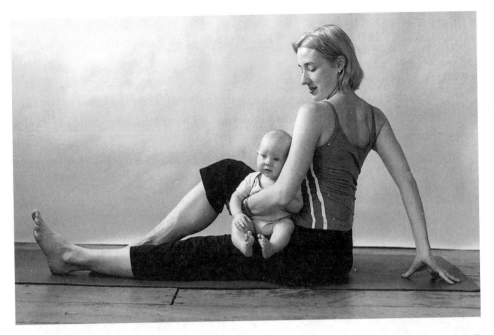

Seated Spinal Twist (with one leg extended)

Essentials

Press the sit bones down and reach the spine up as you spiral around the length of your back.

What if . . .

If it is hard to sit upright with one leg extended, sit on a pillow.

Cool Thing

Because this pose works the muscles of your middle and upper back, it will help relieve neck and shoulder pain.

HEAD TO KNEE POSE *(Janu Sirsasana)*

Mum

- Sit with your legs extended forward. Bend the left knee back and to the side, drawing the knee behind you so that the angle created by your legs is greater than 90 degrees.
- The left foot is relaxed and the left heel is against the inner-left thigh, near your perineum.
- Rotate your abdomen toward the extended leg and stretch your torso and chest over it, keeping your back long.
- If your hands are free, reach toward the extended ankle or foot.
- Keep the knee of the extended leg pointed toward the ceiling and the back of that leg pressed against the mat.
- Repeat on the other side.

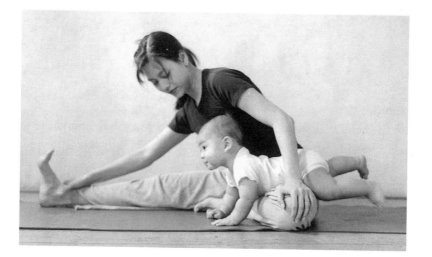

Head to Knee Pose

Baby

Your baby is propped over the thigh of your bent leg, helping to keep your thigh down while she works on her back, neck, and head extension.

Essentials

Think of lining up your navel over the center of your extended thigh. Keep your navel drawn in toward your spine.

What if . . .

If your bent leg or hip comes off the floor, release out of the twist, drop your sit bone, and begin again.

Cool Thing

This *asana* is a great postpartum pose as you reorient your reproductive organs toward your center.

LOCUST POSE *(Salabhasana)*

Mum

- Lie on your stomach with your legs and feet extended behind you, legs together.
- Place your hands on the mat alongside your torso with the palms facing up.
- Press your pubic bone into the mat and lengthen your lower back as you lift your torso and legs off the floor.
- Extend your ankles away from the hips and your head away from your waist.
- Try to lift your shoulders as high as your feet.

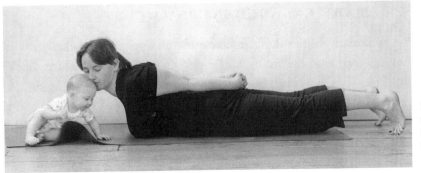

Locust Pose with Chest Opening Variation

Baby

Your baby is lying on her stomach, nose to nose with you: tummy play!

Essentials

Keep your head lifted in line with the slightly arched spine, not dropped forward.

What if . . .

If your legs move apart, lower them a little and draw the inner thighs together. Then try the lift again.

Cool Thing

It's shocking how challenging this can be!

Chest Opening and Leg Variation

- Interlace your hands behind your back and straighten arms.
- Extend your hands away from your shoulders to lift and open your chest. Release.
- Place your hands beneath your head and rest your forehead on them.
- Press your legs together and bend your knees, allowing your feet to face the ceiling.
- Lift your knees and thighs off the mat.

BABY ENGAGEMENT IN LOCUST

As we've said, many babies don't immediately take to tummy play but with encouragement they come around. Interestingly, it is often the more colicky babies who like tummy play, and the mellower babies who don't. Even a disgruntled baby will eventually acclimate, however, and the benefits are well worth the effort. If your baby is protesting being put on his tummy, start with just a few moments and lots of encouragement.

Mum

Sit in any comfortable position.

Baby

Your baby is lying on his belly, facing away from you.

For Baby's Legs

- Gently bend your baby's right knee so that the leg forms a right angle and his foot approaches his buttocks.
- Holding his ankle, make little circles in both directions. Then gently flex and point the foot.
- Release that leg and change sides.
- Lift and extend each leg three times.
- Gently tap his heels together and rub his toes and then the soles of his feet together.

Mum

Lie on your stomach, facing your baby.

For Baby's Arms

- Place your baby on his belly facing you.
- Open your baby's fingers and place his palms on the floor near his shoulders (see page 28).
- If his fingers don't uncurl, use the hand-opening techniques from Baby Engagement (see page 27).
- Soon he will practice pushing against the floor with his hands. He will lift his head to look around.
- Play peek-a-boo while you are working in Locust Pose.

BABY ENGAGEMENT EXERCISE: CRAWLING

- Your baby is on his tummy with his head away from you.
- Place his hands ahead of him on the floor, then gently bend his knees out to the side, bringing his feet in toward his groin one at a time. His whole inner leg will rest on the floor.
- Place your palms against the soles of his feet, giving gentle resistance as he uses them to propel himself forward. You can put a favorite toy ahead of him. As he inches toward it, he will get even more satisfaction from his loco-motion.

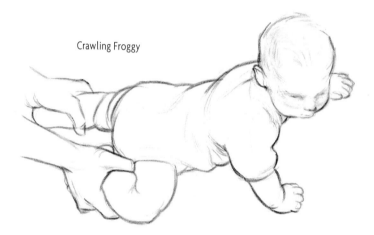

Crawling Froggy

FULL BOW (Dhanurasana)

Mum
- Rest on your belly, legs extended hip-width behind you.
- Bend your knees toward the buttocks and reach behind you to grasp both ankles.
- Lift the head, chest, knees, and thighs off the floor, creating the shape of a bow.
- Press your feet into your hands to lift the head and chest even higher.
- Lift your feet to the same height as your shoulders.

- Press the pubic bone into the floor to maintain space in the lower back.
- Drop your shoulders away from the ears, widen your chest, and let your shoulder blades slide down the back.
- Let your head float upward, not backward.
- Don't let your knees move too far apart. See if the feet can touch, limiting the outward spread of the knees.
- On an exhale, slowly release back down to the ground before letting go of your ankles. Don't let your feet spring out of your hands.
- Rock the hips side to side releasing lower back.
- Press back into Child's Pose to release the back muscles (see page 47).

Baby

Your baby is on his tummy facing you. He may be experimenting with pushing onto all fours with his butt in the air.

Essentials

Press the pubic bone into the floor for support and lift your head, breathing deeply and evenly as you broaden your collarbones. Your breath may even rock you back and forth.

What if . . .

If your knees hurt in this pose, separate the legs wider than hip-width apart.

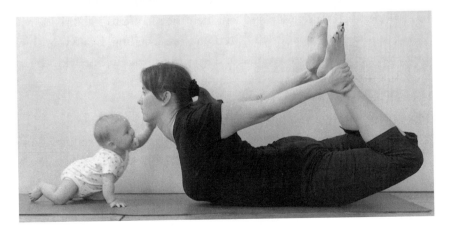

Full Bow

Cool Thing

You and your baby are eye to eye.

Variation—A Little Less Challenging

- Lie flat on your belly as in Full Bow.
- Reach back for one ankle with the same side hand, keeping the other arm and leg extended.
- Press the foot into the hand and lift the thigh and chest off the ground.
- Keep the hips even and the tailbone lengthened toward the pubic bone.
- Keep the extended leg on the ground and use the extended arm to help lift the chest.
- Keep your head in line with the spine.
- Change sides and repeat.
- Try adding a lift of the extended arm and leg off the ground at the same time as the bent leg.

CAMEL POSE (Ustrasana)

Mum

- Kneel with your legs slightly apart, feet flexed and the toes and balls of your feet pressing against the mat. Keep the hips directly over the knees.
- Draw the thigh muscles up and lengthen the sacrum to stabilize your pelvis over your knees as you lift your sternum to the ceiling. Draw your shoulder blades back as the sternum lifts, and keep your head in line with the spine. Look at the ceiling and keep expanding across the chest.
- Reach down behind you to grasp your heels.
- Keep your lower spine long and supported to avoid back strain.
- To release, let your eyes scan forward along the ceiling, leading your head and finally your back into the starting position. Sit on your heels to rest lower back.

Baby

Your baby is lying either in front of you or behind you.

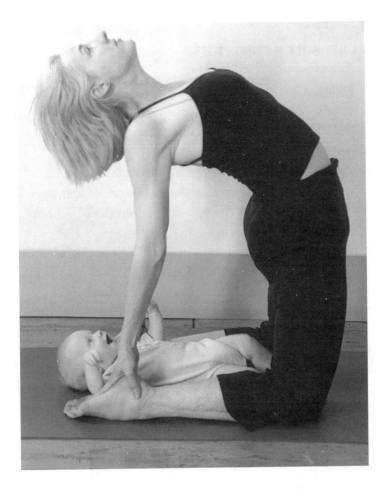

Camel Pose

Essentials
The hips must stay directly over the knees to avoid strain on knee ligaments.

What if . . .
If your lower back hurts, don't bring your hands to your feet. They can begin by resting on your buttocks for support as you arch back. Gradually work into the full position as your lower back and abdomen get stronger and more flexible.

Cool Thing
This pose teaches you to keep your chest open as you use your back muscles.

HALF WHEEL POSE (*Setu Bandhasana*)

Mum

- Lie on your back with your knees bent and feet on the floor close to the sit bones. Inhale and exhale, drawing your navel toward the mat. Your hands are by your sides.
- Keep your knees parallel and press your big toe joint down.
- Keep your collarbones broad and draw your shoulder blades underneath you.
- Press your feet into the mat to lift the hips and roll up through the spine, slowly.
- Think of the hipbones moving toward the ceiling, and the thighs rotating inward.
- Stay up and feel the backs of your legs and gluteal muscles working.
- Roll back down slowly, trying to feel each vertebra as it makes contact with the mat.
- Repeat several times.

Baby

- Your baby is sitting on your abdomen supported by your hands and thighs.

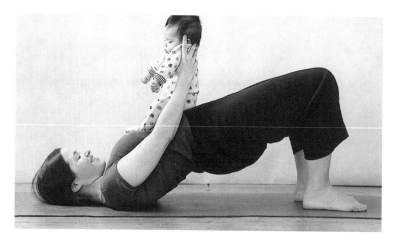

Half
Wheel
Pose
(hips up)

Essentials

Draw your abdomen in toward your spine and lengthen your tailbone so you roll fluidly down your spine and your back does not arch away from the floor.

What if . . .

If your lower back feels strained, press your feet into the floor to help lengthen your back. Do not practice the variations.

Cool Thing

This *asana* feels very comforting.

Variation for Upper Abdominal Strength (for Mum)

- With your back flat on the mat, draw the navel to the spine on an exhale.
- Lift your head and look down your body as you strengthen your upper abdominals.

Variation for Lower Abdominal Strength (for Mum)

- Start with both feet extending to the ceiling; knees can be slightly bent.
- With your whole sacrum in contact with the floor, slowly lower one leg toward the floor; it does not have to touch.
- Slowly raise the lowered leg back up to meet the lifted leg.
- Repeat on the other side. This equals one cycle; repeat five times.

BABY ENGAGEMENT EXERCISES IN HALF WHEEL (*Setu Bandhasana*)

Flying Child Pose II

These exercises for the baby build on the Flying Child Pose I from Class 1. This version has slightly more complex movements and adds new activities for mother and baby. The baby will move through a greater range of space and be taken through a larger variety of activities and play. You will use increased strength in your legs, arms, and torso. This period in your baby's life is a great time for these exercises because he has good head control and is developing the arch of his upper spine and his back. The movements encourage your baby to extend his limbs and it is gratifying to watch him explore his surroundings with increasing confidence.

Mum

Lie on your back with your knees together and folded into your chest and your feet relaxed.

Baby

- Your baby is lying stomach down on your shins held securely by your hands on either side of his rib cage.
- Gently bounce your knees, giving your baby a ride. Use variations like slow and fast, high and low, stopping and starting.
- Bring your knees closer into your chest, and kiss your baby. Repeat three times.
- Extend your legs away from you and back again, giving kisses to your baby on each return.
- Extend your feet toward the ceiling, straightening your legs.
- Your baby will slide down your legs to your abdomen, controlled by your hands. Repeat a few times.

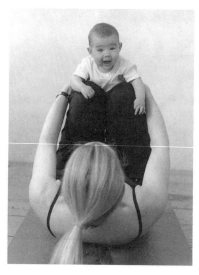

Flying Child

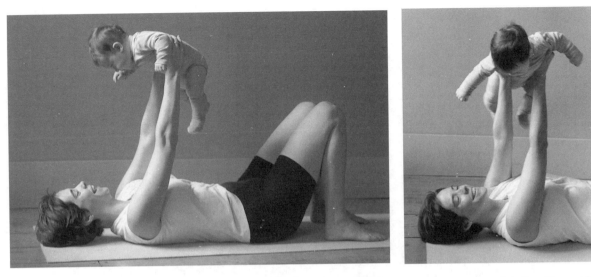

Baby Press

Baby Press (figure-eight)

Baby Press

- While lying on your back, hold your baby around his rib cage and do several baby presses, lifting him up and down above your chest. Keep your shoulder blades in contact with the mat and let your arms do all the work.
- Lower and give lots of kisses.
- On a lift, slowly wave him from side to side, as if you were drawing a figure eight on the ceiling, leading with his head. He's flying!
- Return to center and lower him to your face as you kiss and coo. Repeat.

Baby Canoe Rolls

- From the Baby Press, hug your baby to your chest.
- Imagine your body is a canoe; roll from side to side.

LYING-DOWN TWIST

Mum

- Lie on your back with bent knees and your legs hip-width apart.
- Cross your right knee over your left, wrapping the foot around the ankle. Let the knees slowly release toward your left side until they rest on the mat.
- Keep your knees at waist height and your shoulders even on the mat.

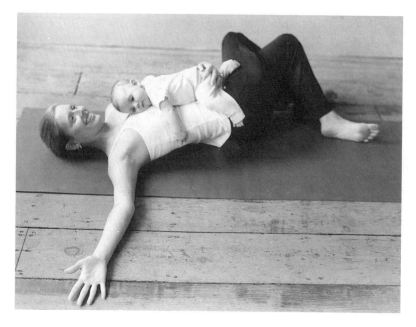

Lying-Down Twist

- This action will roll your pelvis to the left creating a twist in the entire torso.
- As much as you can, stay broad across your chest and keep both shoulders on the mat, letting your belly release as you feel the opposing stretch from right knee through right fingertips.
- Repeat on the other side.

Baby

Your baby can lie or sit on your chest (it gives a nice release to the upper back), or he can sit on your hipbone, encouraging your hip to drop and release.

Essentials

Keep your upper back on the mat and your spine long, deepening the twist.

What if . . .

If one shoulder pops up off the floor, place a pillow underneath your knees.

Cool Thing

This twist can help relieve sciatica and lower back pain and the wrapped leg position may reduce swelling and possibly even varicose veins in the legs.

RESTING POSE (*Savasana*)

With supported knees.

Mum

- Lie on your back, placing a large pillow beneath your knees.
- If your knees splay to the side, do not let them fall off the pillow.
- Completely relax the weight of your body into the floor.
- Focus your mind on your exhalation, following it to its end. This will naturally slow your breathing.

Baby

Your baby can lie on you, chest to chest, nursing, or she may lie by your side.

Essentials
Let everything release as your body absorbs the benefits of the poses you have done.

What if . . .
If your lower back feels strained, prop knees up higher.

Cool Thing
You may actually take a cat nap in this pose. Many yoga teachers feel that *savasana* is the most important pose in *asana* practice.

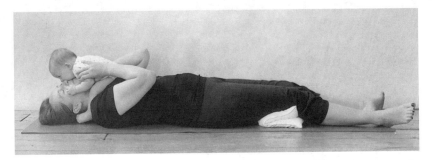

Resting Pose (knees on cushion)

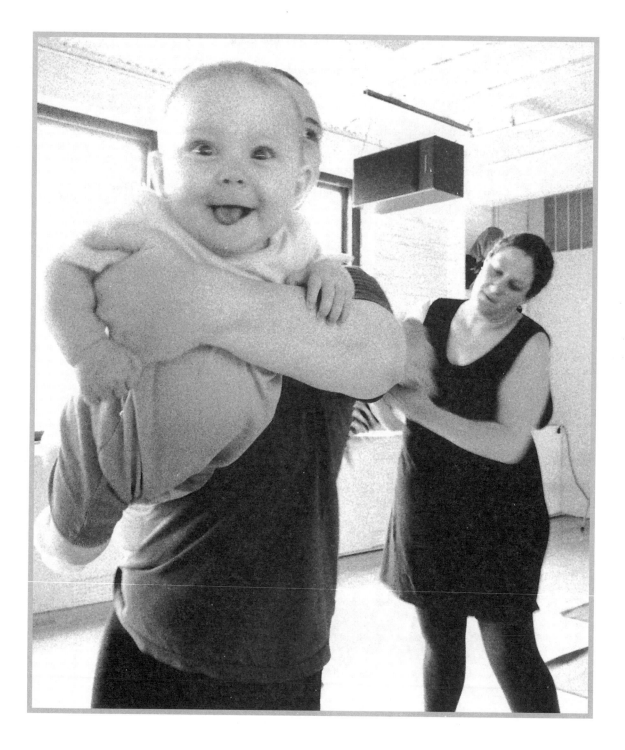

6

CLASS 3:
Six to Twelve Months

A CLASS FOR ASSIMILATION

APPROXIMATELY 45 MINUTES; HOLD EACH POSE FOR FIVE TO EIGHT BREATHS.

Breathing Exercise: Segmented Breathing

Sitting Pose

Revolved Wide-Leg Stretch

Modified and Full Boat Pose with Roll

Sun Salute, Series III

Triangle Pose

Extended Angle Pose

Revolved Triangle Pose

Preparation for Handstand and Full Handstand

Cow Facing Pose

Gate Pose

Cobra

Full Bow

Half Wheel Pose with Variations

Revolved Belly Pose

Bound Angle Pose

Seated Forward Bend

Resting Pose

Multitasking is a word that entered the language fairly recently, but mothers or caretakers of young children have known for centuries that shortly after birth you need to learn how to do several things at once, and you need to acquire this skill quickly. Multitasking is needed to pay the electric bill, clean up cracker crumbs, and finish getting dressed, while making sure the baby doesn't swallow the tiny Lego pieces her older brother left on the floor. By age six months and beyond, everyone is branching out.

Class 3 is challenging. We have designed it so that you can really use your body and energy in a way you may not have been able to previously. It has an expansive quality which we've found mothers love at this point. Your ability to do more corresponds to your baby's increased mobility as she crawls, cruises, or even walks. Just as your baby is becoming intrigued by the greater accessibility of the world, you too are beginning to realize a renewed sense of mobility. After months of feeling confined by a variety of physical restrictions—both yours and your baby's—the increased range of possibilities will seem miraculous to both of you.

Your baby is now benefiting more from floor play, so the two of you can become a yoga team. She will have her own way of interacting with you. This is the beginning of a beautiful, unique, and complicated relationship. We created this class with that in mind. The poses here become more challenging, requiring more effort but delivering increased strength as you move through them. These *asanas* energize and open the body. Breathe deeply and enjoy yourself.

Your baby may now be more physically engaged, using your standing poses as a cruising aid and your seated poses as an obstacle course. She may even crawl on your back in Forward Bends and help you deepen the pose just a bit more. Alternatively, she may want to gnaw at your toes as you practice the partnering work as in the Seated Forward Bend. Laura's son, Dylan, liked to grab her nose and bite it affectionately every time her face came near him. Whatever the relationship, remember that all this activity is valuable bonding time for you and your baby. Yoga has its serious side, but it should also be fun for the two of you, a period of the day you both look forward to.

The Class

Class 3 brings together elements of each of the other classes, drawing from their specific qualities to create a class with enough variety to be challenging during this period. The Sun Salute series is fun and stimulating enough to create the heat necessary to move deeply into the poses that follow. The standing poses are held longer, which is great for developing strength and stamina, and also allows your body to fully experience the benefits of each pose. We have included some more advanced twists, such as the Revolved Triangle and the Revolved Belly poses. These continue to work on the abdominal area with the internal massage and increased circulation they deliver. Poses such as Extended Angle and Gate feel fabulous and tone and lengthen the waist. The Full Wheel is a pose not everyone will do. It feels wonderful, and nothing beats it for reversing rounded shoulders and general slouching, but if you have had a diastasis (a weakening of the connective tissue in the abdominal wall) you should be cautious, and if your shoulders are particularly stiff it will be difficult to place your hands correctly. The Half Wheel series is even more playful; feel free to add old or new variations. Each pose builds on or provides counterstretch to the last. This balanced class can be done from six to twelve months and beyond. It can form the core of your practice for as long as you want. Enjoy!

Your Body

At 6–12 months postpartum some women feel completely restored to their former selves; others are at least starting to feel that way. There may be a predictable routine to your child's sleep patterns, and you may have established a few routines that work for you as well. A sense of proportion and logic is returning to your life.

It is also at this point that habitual postural adjustments are making themselves known; for instance, if you always carry your daughter on one hip (now that she is able to hold herself upright) or talk on the phone by cradling the receiver between one shoulder and your ear to free up your hands, you may be feeling a lateral pull in the spine or a kink in the phone shoulder. This is when left- or right-sidedness takes a toll on our body. As an experiment, try reversing your patterns: hold your baby on the other hip, hold the phone in the other hand. It will probably feel strange, but the increasing weight of your baby is something to contend with now and will exacerbate problems that arise from these physical habits. Whether you are twisting and lifting, carrying a stroller down subway steps, or hoisting a car seat in and out of the backseat, be aware of how you are doing these things. Each one-sided movement deserves an opposing movement. This doesn't usually happen naturally in life, so it is important to use your yoga class to encourage a neutral balance in your body, evening out the right and left sides.

A collapsed posture is insidious. So many tasks in your life seem to be conspiring to foist it upon you. Even dancers and yogis are susceptible. Yoga teacher Donna Farhi says that when the heart and chest are sunken downward, one's whole outlook will follow a dispirited path. Despite everything, from gravity to your child pulling at you, do the best you can to resist this posture.

You and your baby may not yet be sleeping through the night. If you can do the prescribed napping while your baby sleeps, good for you, but if you can't catch up on sleep during these brief respites, remind yourself that you are doing more than you ever have before. No doubt you are doing everything you used to do (possibly working a full- or part-time job) plus nursing and caring for another human being at the same time. A long slow breath and a few chest-opening poses will help when you feel overwhelmed.

This is a good time to assess the progress you've made and to consider any problem areas you want to work on. You may be wondering if the extra kilos will ever depart, or if you have now met your permanent new body. Give yourself more time, and above all, don't be hard on yourself. Concentrate on the idea that your muscles are becoming stronger and your alignment is improving, and you'll feel more capable each time you do a class. We used to talk after every session about the new ground regained, each time realizing that this must have been what we felt like before. One of our students, Tina, a dancer from a major modern dance company, regained her considerable strength quickly, but even through her sixth and seventh postpartum month she would groan every time we did poses requiring upper-body strength. By month ten, however, she was holding Plank Pose with the best of them. Whatever your particular concern, remember that you are taking steps toward your future goals.

Your Baby

Class 3 covers a longer time span, 6–12 months. You are the center of your child's world now, and she craves your loving and playful care. Developmental changes are starting to happen at an accelerated pace. Teeth are coming in, and your baby's mood reflects the discomfort she feels as gums erupt. She may be sitting up, but not all that steadily, so you are on call to prevent a spill at any moment. Once your child achieves a basic degree of confidence, she will begin to crawl and then to cruise. Each skill comes with its own set of assurances and insecurities. As your baby pushes off from the dock of your complete assistance, you will find each small accomplishment incredible and endlessly fascinating.

Your baby is now working hard at perfecting the skills she has already achieved, as well as expanding her repertoire. The neck and back strength she has been developing will now be useful to keep her vertical when sitting up. The arm strength gained from pushing up into Cobra will help as she raises herself onto all fours to prepare for crawling, or uses her arms as props to balance in a seated position. Before she could crawl, Sarah's daughter, Rosey, like many babies, did an amazing Downward Facing Dog. This position is good for arm strength and prepares babies for crawling as they evolve from a quadruped to a biped. When crawling, babies use opposing arms and legs, a coordination that these exercises help develop. They may still be working on rolling from stomach to back, or the more difficult back to stomach, using their hands, an important aid to locomotion. Most children will want to stand at around six months but cannot support their own weight and will need your hands for guidance.

On the fine motor skill front, they will be working on reaching and grabbing, starting to grasp with pointer finger and thumb. Children are constantly picking up and letting go of things. Rosey liked to pinch painted toenails. They clap and can play hand games. By nine to ten months of age they will want to practice pulling up to a standing position for long stretches of time. At about this time they may begin to cruise on their own, maybe even while holding on to your leg as you do standing poses. They have so many new skills and want to use them all. The exercises in Class 3 work toward increased movement in space with larger and more complicated movements. Your baby is on her way to upright mobility. Babies of this age love to play peek-a-boo, flirting with separation, and they adore your coming and going as you swan-dive in the Sun Salute series. The baby-engagement rolling exercise we did in Class 2, which encouraged the single roll, now becomes a multiple roll down your legs and back again. Doing yoga with babies at this age is great fun. Your baby will love to watch you in motion, involved in an activity that revolves around her.

BREATHING EXERCISE:
SEGMENTED BREATHING

This breathing exercise is particularly useful for quieting your racing mind. As with all of the breathing practices it can be done in a seated or reclining position; however, we recommend you start with this one in *savasana* (Resting Pose) because the exercise is more complex and requires some breath retention. Your body should be relaxed and your mind focused on the breath. When inhaling, think of sipping the air rather than gulping. When exhaling, think of a long even release of air rather than a rush. If you need to take a regular breath in between cycles, go ahead, then return to the pattern. Imagine that you fill first your belly and then your chest with air as you draw the breath in.

- Start lying down, with a pillow under your back (see Supine Chest Opener, page 178).
- Let your body relax and your eyes and throat soften.
- Exhale completely through your nose. When you exhale, let the breath slip out in a slow measured way.
- Inhale through your nose for a count of two. Do not attempt to fill the lungs completely. Pause for a count of two.
- Inhale for another two counts and pause for two. Your breath is rising higher in your chest.
- Inhale for another count of two and pause for two. Now your lungs are full.
- Exhale completely.
- Repeat for five full cycles (three short inhales and a complete exhale is a cycle).
- Breathe normally for a few breaths or anytime you need a break during the exercise.

SITTING POSE *(Siddhasana)*

Mum

- Start in a cross-legged sitting position.
- Lift your chest and broaden across your collarbones.
- Feel your weight evenly distributed into both sit bones.
- Release your shoulder blades down your back.
- Lengthen your spine from the tailbone to the top of your head.
- Inhale through your nose and on the exhale, chant *Om* to your baby.
- After finishing your *Om*(s), practice your Kegels.

Baby

Your baby can either sit in your lap or lie on the floor in front of you. Make contact with your baby through touch, gaze, or sound.

Essentials

Find a moment of stillness before your active practice.

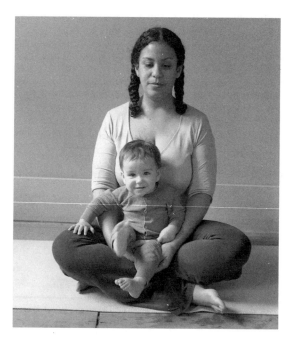

Sitting Pose

What if . . .

If it's hard to sit up straight, sit on a pillow.

Cool Thing

This pose makes you feel very peaceful!

Variation to Warm Up Spine

- Sit in *siddhasana*.
- Move the left arm overhead and lean to the right.
- The shoulder blades move down your back as you stretch to the right side.
- Lift your body up through center then lower to the left, right arm overhead.
- Come back up, repeat the first side, and instead of coming up through center, sweep the left arm and torso forward and around to the left, and reach right arm up to left.
- Repeat each variation four times.

REVOLVED WIDE-LEG STRETCH *(Upavistha Konasana)*

Mum

- Sit with your legs open in a wide V, legs straight and knees and toes pointing toward the ceiling.

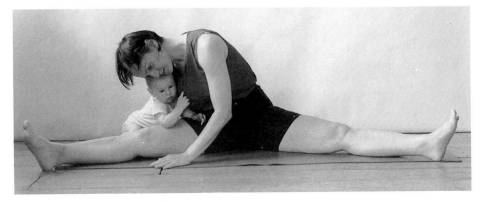

Revolved Wide-Leg Stretch

- Rotate the torso and bring your hands to either side of the right leg.
- Extend the spine and feel even weight in each sit bone.
- Press your left hip down into the mat as you turn right, rotating both sides of the rib cage toward the leg.
- Bend over the right leg, aiming your navel over the center of your right thigh and your sternum toward the ankle.
- Walk your arms alongside the leg. Feel the sides of your spine getting longer and more even as you deepen the bend; keep the front of your body extended.
- Release your abdomen and hips.
- Inhale as you come up and repeat to other side.

Baby

You may place your baby across your free leg, his chest on your thigh, his arms reaching for the floor, as you extend your torso. His weight will help you keep the back of your thigh on the floor as he works his upper-body strength. Or, place your baby on the inside of the leg you will be extending over. Tickle and coo as you move toward his face.

Essentials
Keep your spine long, and both sit bones pressing into the mat.

What if . . .
If your lower back rounds in this pose, sit on a pillow to lift your hips slightly.

Cool Thing
The more you can relax your stomach, the deeper the twist.

MODIFIED AND FULL BOAT POSE (Navasana)

Mum
- Sit on the mat with your knees bent and feet on the floor.
- Hold your outer thighs and lift your chest.

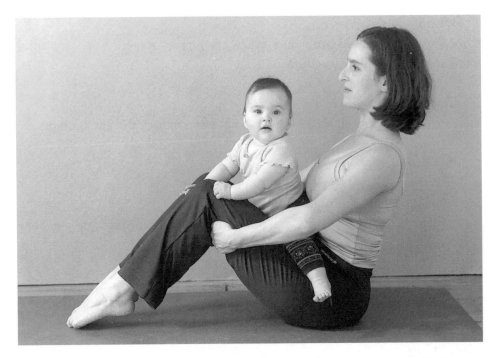

Modified Boat Pose

- Keeping your abdominal muscles engaged and chest lifted, raise your feet just off the floor.
- Let your torso tilt back slightly for balance and keep your lower back moving up and in.
- If you can, raise your shins so that they are parallel to the floor and reach your hands toward your feet.
- Straighten your legs so you create a large V shape (Full Boat).

Baby

Baby is on your lap facing away from you. If your hands are free, stretch your arms toward your shins with the palms facing in. To rest, extend your legs along the mat and move your torso into a Forward Bend and kiss your baby.

Essentials

Your lower back must remain lifted.

What if . . .

If you feel as though you are falling backward, support yourself with your arms, palms on the floor behind your hips.

Cool Thing

This is really great for your abdomen and spine, and your baby will *love* the motion.

Roll Variation

- Your baby is lying on your shins, stomach down.
- Hold your baby's rib cage.
- Curve your lower back and roll down through the spine bringing your baby with you.
- Try to kiss your baby as you roll down.
- Use your abdominal muscles and the weight of your baby, initiating a return to a seated position.
- Repeat five times.

BABY ENGAGEMENT IN BOAT POSE

In this class, the babies have graduated to sitting on your lap for the baby exercises. During the second six months of life your baby may be eager to test her independence. At first, she may not be able to sit unassisted, but soon enough she will be. Practice these exercises in front of a mirror from time to time. Babies really enjoy looking at their own reflection. Many of these exercises are new; some are variations of ones you have done before.

Baby

Sit with your legs extended in front of you. Your baby is sitting in your lap.

For Baby's Arms: Open-and-Close Hands with Variations

- Hold your baby's hands and gently start to open and close them.
- You can cross her arms over each other (alternating which arm is on top) and add clapping for rhythmic variation.

- Wheel her hands 'round and 'round each other (like "the wheels on the bus") then bring her hands to her tummy, walk them up her torso to her mouth, and help her blow big kisses.
- Have your baby experiment with touching her own face, ears, nose, and cheeks.
- Still holding her hands, lean back slightly, extending her arms up as her back rests against your stomach.
- Circle her arms from the same position. Reverse the direction of circles.
- Move her arms up and down, up and down.

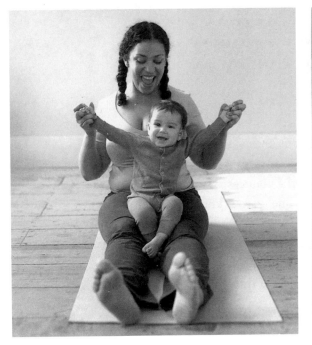

Baby's arms open

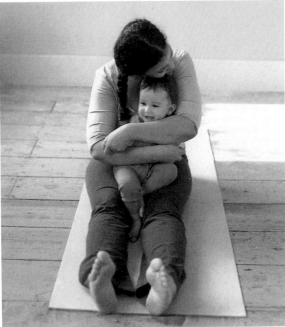

Baby's arms closed

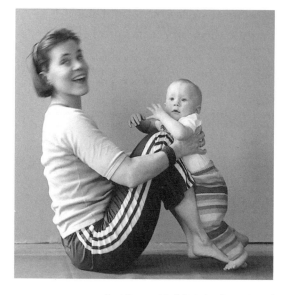

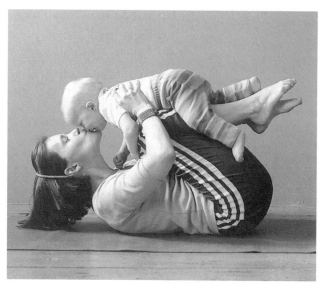

Boat Pose and Roll Variation (mum sitting)

Boat Pose and Roll Variation (mum on back)

BABY SITTING ON THIGHS: FACING OUT OR IN

Baby

- Your baby is sitting on your thighs.
- Holding him at the waist, bounce your knees (and your baby) in a rhythm, then stop intermittently. He will wait in suspense for the surprise interruptions. Play with the speed and size of the bounces.
- Still holding him at the waist, raise one of your knees and then the other, tilting him from side to side.
- With your baby sitting on your knees, keep your knees together and walk your feet in toward your hips. Your knees and baby will rise. Gently let your feet slide forward for a surprise drop. Repeat three times.

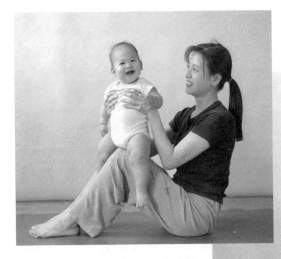

Baby Variation (up)

Baby Variation (down)

- Walk your knees in again, this time leaning your baby from side to side before the surprise drop.

Standing to Kneeling

Support your baby in a standing position. Hold him around his rib cage and easily lean him toward you. He will resist bending his knees at first, but will soon learn to do it. This is an important tool for him to have when he finds himself standing solo and unable to come down.

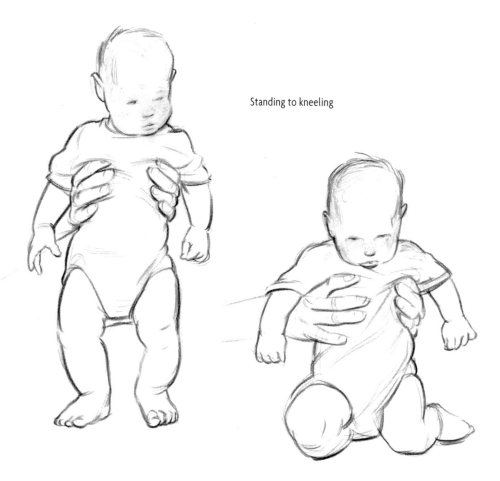

Standing to kneeling

BABY FLIPS

Baby

- Sit with your legs together in front of you, knees comfortably bent and touching, and feet on the floor.
- Place your baby in the crease of your hips, facing you.
- Gently take hold of your baby's hips, with your fingers on her belly and thumbs on her bum.
- Lift her up and turn her upside down until her belly comes to rest on your bent knees and thighs. She will probably push against your legs with her arms in order to see you.

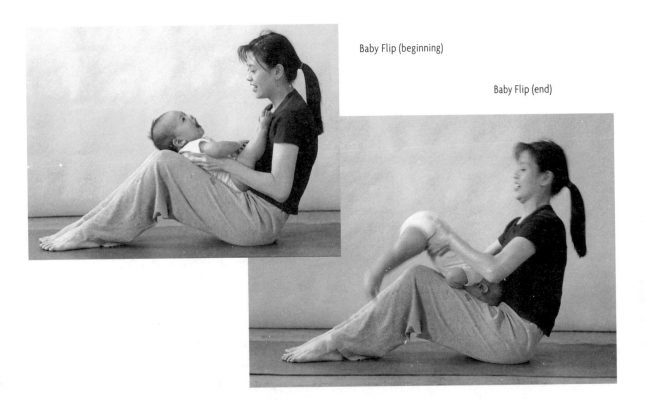

Baby Flip (beginning)

Baby Flip (end)

- Lower your knees and congratulate her on her flips.
- Repeat. If your legs are not comfortable, sitting on a bed will be fine.

SUN SALUTE, SERIES III *(Surya Namaskar)*

This is another of the classic Sun Salute series, which provides a complete warm-up and increases both strength and flexibility. Stand with your feet baby width or narrower, as you begin to return to your pre-pregnancy stance.

MOUNTAIN POSE *(Tadasana)*

- Stand with feet baby-width apart or narrower.
- Inhale, your arms overhead with the palms together.

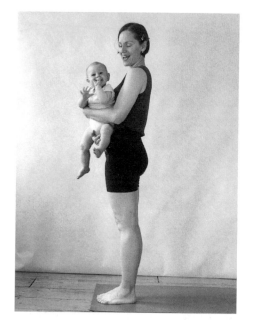

Mountain Pose

FORWARD BEND (*Uttanasana*) AND LUNGE

- Exhale and bend forward over straight legs with an extended spine. The front of your body should remain very long, and your abdomen should be relaxed.
- Inhale and step your right leg straight behind you into a Lunge.
- Exhale and stretch the front of your thigh, letting your pelvis move toward the floor.

DOWNWARD FACING DOG (*Adho Mukha Svanasana*)

- Inhale in Lunge and exhale, stepping your left foot back to the right, raising your hips into Downward Facing Dog.
- Your feet should be slightly wider than hip-width apart, with your pelvis floating up toward the ceiling, your kneecaps lifted, and your heels moving back and down. Hold this pose for five full breaths.
- Keep your navel drawn in toward your spine to engage your abdominal muscles.

PLANK

- From Downward Facing Dog, inhale and move your torso forward until your body is in one long, extended line, like a push-up.
- Push from the balls of your feet.

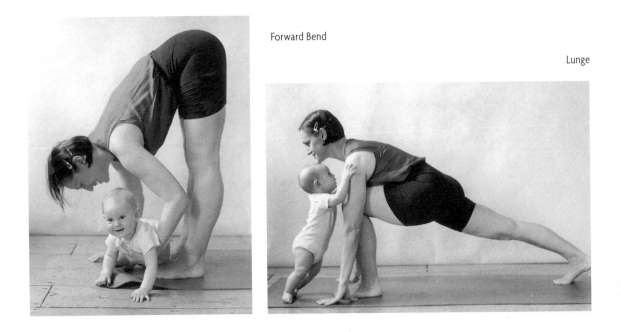

Forward Bend

Lunge

FOUR-LEGGED STICK POSE VARIATION (*Mini-Chaturanga*)

- Exhale and place your knees on the mat, pressing your bent elbows into your sides and holding your torso a few centimeters above floor. Keep the hips in line with the body.
- Make sure shoulders don't round forward. Keep your head in line with the shoulders.

UPWARD FACING DOG (*Urdhva Mukha Svanasana*)

- Inhale and slide forward with your torso, straightening your arms and legs and suspending your outstretched body slightly off the floor using your hands and tops of the feet. Your shoulders should be directly over your wrists and relaxed, away from your ears.
- Alternatively, you can extend into Cobra (see page 152), keeping your legs on the mat and torso arching up, supported by your hands.

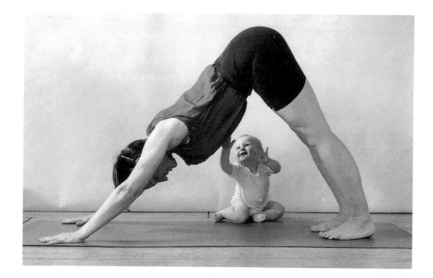

Downward Facing Dog

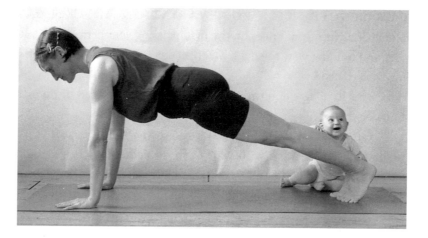

Plank

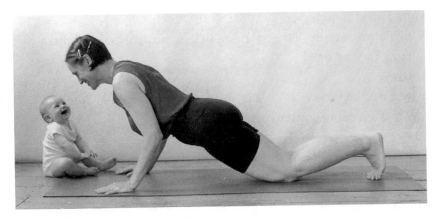

Mini-Chaturanga

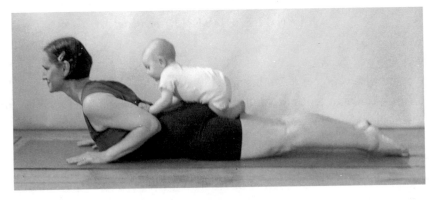

Cobra

To Finish

Downward Facing Dog (*Adho Mukha Svanasana*)
Exhale into Downward Facing Dog.

Lunge
From Downward Facing Dog, inhale and move your right leg next to your right hand. Your left extends back. Exhale.

Forward Bend (*Uttanasana*)

- Inhale, and step the left leg forward to join the right and straighten your legs into a Forward Bend.
- Exhale.
- Inhale and reverse swan-dive up into *tadasana* (Mountain Pose).
- Exhale your arms down to your sides.

Repeat the entire sequence on the other side with the left leg stepping to lunge. Do the series two to four times.

TRIANGLE POSE (*Trikonasana*)

Mum

- Stand with your feet 1.2 to 1.5 meters apart.
- Turn your right foot out 90 degrees and turn left toes in slightly. The front heel should line up with the arch of the back foot.
- Reach both arms out to the side at shoulder height.
- Lift your waist and torso evenly and extend your spine long.
- Keep length in the sides of the torso as you extend your torso sideways over your right leg. Keep your hips facing forward.
- Place your right hand on your shin and reach your left hand straight up toward the ceiling.
- Repeat on the other side.

Baby

Position your baby alongside the foot you will be stretching toward. (When you change sides, bring the other foot next to your baby). He will love to see you turn yourself into a mobile as you circle your arm.

Essentials

Do not let your torso lean forward or backward. Stay in line with your legs as though you were two-dimensional, or between two panes of glass.

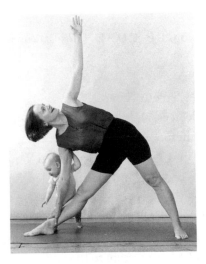

Triangle Pose

What if . . .

If you feel a collapse or jamming in the front leg, vigorously lift both sides of the kneecap. You may also think of the shin as moving forward as the thigh moves back.

Cool Thing

Triangle pose always feels good.

Arm Circle Variation

- Move the top arm in a big circle starting over the head, past your baby, along the body, and around again. Tickle your baby as you pass by. Do this three times.
- Repeat on the other side.

EXTENDED ANGLE POSE *(Parsvakonasana)*

Mum

- Stand with your feet 1.2 to 1.5 meters apart.
- Turn your left foot out 90 degrees, and turn right toes in slightly.
- Press the outside of your right foot into the ground.
- Slowly bend your left knee into a right angle (just as in Warrior II).
- Extend your torso over the bent leg and place your left forearm on the left thigh.
- Keep your chest wide and shoulder blades dropped down your back.
- Keep your pelvis and torso facing forward and your spine long.
- Imagine a long, extended line from sacrum to head.
- Extend your right arm overhead on a long diagonal from heel to the fingertips.
- To assume the complete position, remove your forearm from your thigh and place your left hand on the floor behind your front foot.
- Circle your right arm, tickling your baby as you pass by.
- Repeat on the other side.

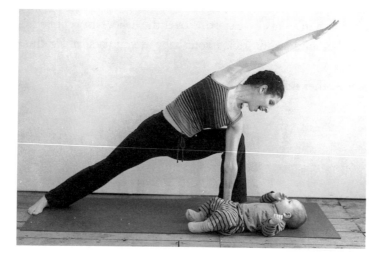

Extended
Angle Pose

Baby

Your baby can rest on the floor next to your front foot and can try to catch your fingers as they circle past.

Essentials

Keep the pelvis open by opening the top hip and ribs toward the ceiling.

What if . . .

If your torso collapses downward, don't go into the full version. Instead, rotate your rib cage toward the ceiling, lengthening both sides of the waist evenly, and keep your forearm on your thigh.

Cool Thing

The side stretch feels great, and you'll feel lighter and breathe more easily after this stretch.

Full Pose Variation

- Instead of placing your arm on your thigh, place your hand on the floor.
- First, place your hand on the *inside* of your foot—use the pressure of the arm to the inner thigh and knee to open your chest to the ceiling.
- Then, change the placement of your hand to the *outside* of your foot—maintain the opened chest and reach a little farther through the upper arm.
- Your upper arm creates an extension of the line of the legs.

REVOLVED TRIANGLE POSE *(Parivrtta Trikonasana)*

Mum

- Stand with your feet about 1.2 meters apart.
- Turn your left foot out 90 degrees, and turn right toes in slightly.
- Place your hands on your waist and square your hips to face the right foot.
- Press down through the feet and keep your weight evenly distributed.
- Bend your torso forward and with an extended back, stretch over the left leg. It may help to think about moving your left hip backward away from you.

- Keeping your spine long, rotate your torso clockwise on an axis from tail to head.
- Your right hand may be on the floor, your ankle, or your shin.
- Extend your left arm up toward the ceiling if you can maintain the open width across the chest, or leave the left hand on the left hip and work on opening your chest.
- Keep your chest wide and your back open.
- Repeat on the other side.

Baby
Your baby can be lying down, sitting, or pulling up on your legs.

Essentials
Hips must be parallel to floor so the spine can extend evenly.

What if . . .
If your top shoulder is unable to rotate, lift your body by placing the right hand higher on your left leg.

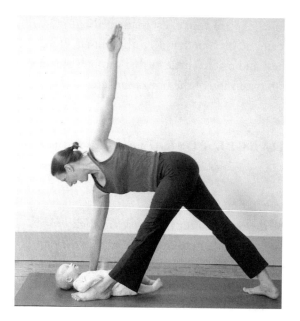

Revolved Triangle Pose

Cool Thing

Twists really do tone the abdomen. They'll continue to improve the "soft belly" of the postnatal body.

PREPARATION FOR HANDSTAND

Mum

- Stand facing the wall, feet hip-width apart.
- Press the palms of the hands against the wall at hip level, fingers toward the ceiling.
- Slowly walk your feet back, keeping your hands on the wall until your torso and arms are fully extended and parallel to the floor.
- Imagine you are reaching your sit bones away from your hands on the wall.
- Head is in line with your arms.
- Keep the legs parallel and very straight, kneecaps lifted.

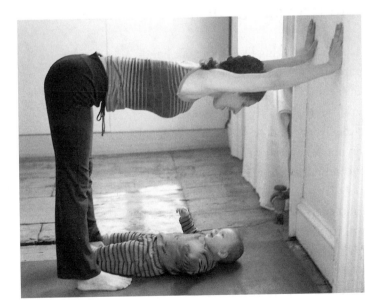

Preparation for Handstand

- Lengthen the lower abdomen up. You can think of your uterus moving back toward your sit bones.
- Step one foot forward to come out of it.

Baby
Your baby is on the floor looking up at you.

Essentials
Do not let your front ribs poke out.

What if . . .
If you are very tight in either your hamstrings or shoulders, walk your hands up the wall and work there until it becomes easier.

Cool Thing
You will still extend your spine, stretching from wrist to hip. You are making a bridge for your baby to crawl under as you stretch from hand to hip.

FULL HANDSTAND (Adho Mukha Vrksasana)

- Start in Downward Facing Dog with your hands 7 centimeters from the wall and your fingers pointing to the wall.
- Walk your feet in closer to your hands.
- Keep your shoulders directly over your wrists.
- Look between your hands at the floor or your baby.
- Straighten one leg and slightly bend the other, preparing to kick up.
- Take a few preliminary hops using the straight leg to swing toward the ceiling and the bent leg to push off the floor.
- Keeping shoulders over your wrists, kick up and reach the straight leg's heel for the wall (the bent leg will follow).
- With both heels on the wall, press the floor away under your hands and reach your feet for the sky.
- Reach the tailbone for the heels and stretch the waist long.
- Hold for a few breaths.

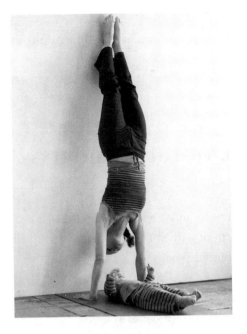

Full Handstand

- Come down by reaching one foot for the floor. Once both feet are down, *slowly* roll up to standing.
- Congratulations! Next time try kicking up with the other leg.

Baby

If you feel very confident in your handstand practice, your baby can lie between your hands; otherwise you can let her have your whole mat to herself, away from you, as you practice against the wall.

Essentials

Your arms must remain straight from wrist to shoulder.

What if . . .

If your arms don't feel strong enough to hold you, practice holding Downward Facing Dog and moving directly to Plank, holding each for longer periods of time to build strength.

Cool Thing

It feels fantastic to be completely upside-down, and standing on your hands (for a change).

COW FACING POSE (GOMUKHASANA)

Mum

- Kneel with your knees crossed and stacked on top of each other, right over left. You may want to start out with your weight supported by your arms and your hands on the mat alongside you.
- Sit between your feet.
- Your left foot is near your right hip, and your right foot is near your left hip.
- Sit with your weight even on both sit bones and hips.

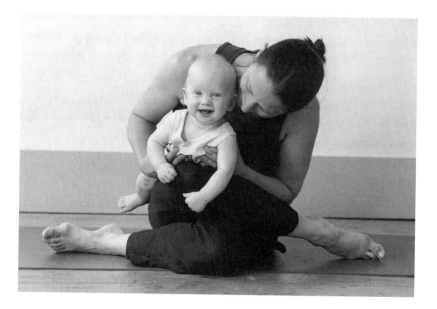

Cow Facing Pose

- Let your hips relax.
- Sit with the spine lifted and collarbones open. Your shoulder blades should be dropped down your back.
- Just sitting here may be enough, but if possible bend your torso forward, keeping the front and back of your body long and your abdomen soft.

Baby

Your baby is sitting in your lap, possibly even imitating your interesting shape.

Essentials

Keep spine lifted and pelvis dropped.

What if . . .

If this is really easy for you, extend your shins away from your hips. Ideally, your shins will be in line with your knees, but it takes *very* open hips to accomplish this.

Cool Thing

It's a great nursing pose.

Arm Variation if You Have Free Hands

- Bring your right hand around to your back with the palm facing out. Bend the elbow and slide your hand up the spine.
- Raise your left arm toward the ceiling and bend the elbow so that your hand reaches behind your head. Let the elbow extend straight up.
- If your hands meet, clasp your fingers together. Or let the fingers of both hands touch.
- Keep your collarbones wide and even.
- Extend your torso forward over the legs.

GATE POSE (*Parighasana*)

Mum

- Start in a kneeling position, with your hips over knees and torso over hips.
- Straighten your right leg to the side, keeping your foot in line with your left knee.
- Lift the torso, lengthening the waist, and keep your hips directly over the bent knee.
- Bending at the hip, reach the torso sideways over the straight leg. Your right hand will rest on your right shin as the left reaches overhead toward your right foot.

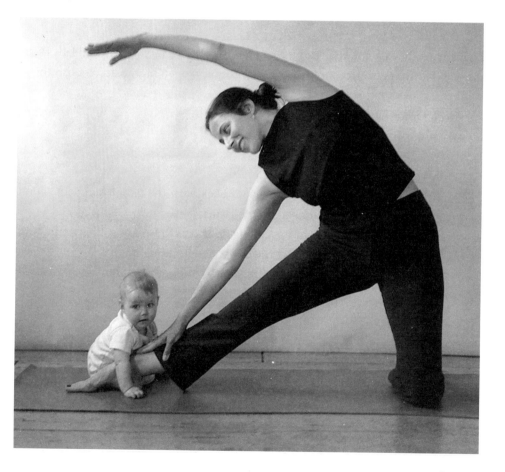

Gate Pose

- Keep your tailbone and sacrum moving in.
- Extend both sides of the waist evenly.
- Take an extra deep breath here while your ribs are fully extended.

Baby

Your baby can sit on your extended leg, facing the foot supported by the bottom arm, or rest on the floor in front of your bent knee.

Essentials

Don't let all the weight shift toward the extended leg. Maintain your center and stretch from there.

What if . . .

If it hurts to kneel, put a blanket under your knees for padding.

Cool Thing

This pose really does help the upper body feel lighter and more open.

COBRA (Bhujangasana I)

Mum

- Lie on your stomach extending your legs straight.
- Bend your elbows and place your palms on the floor alongside your shoulders, directly under your armpits.
- Press into your hands as you extend your spine up into a forward arc. Imagine you are pulling yourself forward.
- Lengthen the sacrum down toward the pubic bone and press into the mat.
- Reach through the legs.
- Extend your sternum forward and inhale as you reach your chest up and toward your baby.
- Release your shoulders away from your ears and move the shoulder blades together down the back.

Baby

Your baby is lying on his stomach facing you, nose to nose.

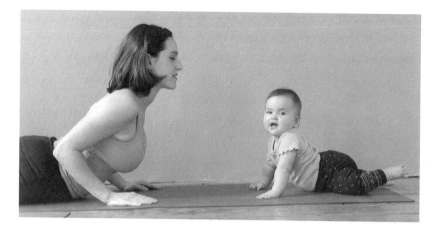

Cobra

Essentials
Your shoulders must move down, away from your ears.

What if . . .
If your lower back hurts, lower your torso, press your pubic bone into the mat, and lengthen your spine in both directions.

Cool Thing
You're doing the same thing as your baby!

BABY ENGAGEMENT IN COBRA

During this period, your baby may be rolling and pushing onto all fours like a little gymnast or he may be content with the quieter pursuits of tummy time. You can easily make tummy time a game when you are lying face to face pushing up into identical Cobras, or you can roll and imitate his variations, especially the perfect arc he creates as he lifts his head up and back. He may experience a certain amount of frustration as he sees an object he wants but can't quite get to it, and may even end up moving himself farther from his objective as he executes a reverse crawl. Being on the yoga mat helps him, though. Instead of sliding, he will get purchase with his toes, helping him to move forward. During this time another cool feat you might see is a baby Downward Facing Dog or Plank move.

Mum

Lie on your stomach facing your baby.

Baby

- Your baby is on his stomach facing you with the full palm of his hand on the floor near his shoulders.
- Come close, so the two of you are nose to nose, and move into Cobra. Repeat three times.
- Play peek-a-boo as you move face to face.
- If your baby is crawling, see if he can sit on your back. This is a fun ride and new view for him.

KNEE CRAWLING

Mum kneels with her baby tummy-down on her lap. Bring your baby's upper body forward enough so that she supports her own weight on her hands. Holding her hips, slowly move with her as she inches her hands forward. This helps her to build arm strength and to have the experience of moving forward rather than that frustrating backward crawl.

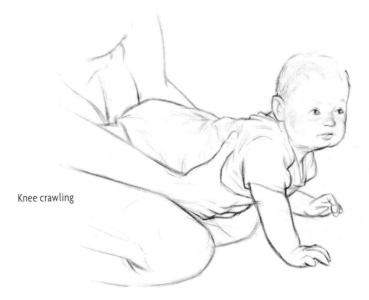

Knee crawling

FULL BOW (*Dhanurasana*)

Mum

- Lie on your stomach with your feet about hip-width apart.
- Bend your knees toward the buttocks and reach behind you to grasp both ankles.
- Lift your head, chest, knees, and thighs off the floor; think of the knees extending away from the hips.
- Press your feet away from you to lift your head and chest even higher.
- Your feet should be at the same height as your shoulders.
- Press the pubic bone into the mat to extend the lower back. Your shoulders should drop away from your ears and your chest should remain wide.
- Let your head float upward not backward.
- Keep your legs parallel and hip-width apart.
- Slowly release back down to the ground before letting go of your ankles. As you release the feet, don't let them spring from your hands.
- Rock your hips from side to side to release the lower back.

Baby

Your baby is lying on her tummy, facing you. She may be experimenting with pushing onto all fours, with her bottom in the air.

Full Bow

Essentials

Press the pubic bone into the mat and lift the head, breathing into your chest as you broaden across the collarbones.

What if . . .

If your knees hurt, separate the legs wider than hip-width apart.

Cool Thing

Though strenuous, this pose can feel quite playful. Try letting your breath rock you back and forth.

HALF WHEEL POSE *(Setu Bandhasana)*

Mum

- Lie on your back with your knees bent and feet on the floor close to the sit bones. Inhale and exhale bringing the navel toward the floor.
- Keep your knees parallel and press your big toe down.
- Keep your collarbones open and draw the shoulder blades together underneath you, arms by your side.
- Press your feet into the ground to lift your hips and roll up through the spine slowly.
- Stretch your pelvis toward the ceiling.
- Roll back down, trying to feel each vertebra of the spine as it makes contact with the mat.
- Repeat several times.
- On the last time, stay up for several breaths and feel the backs of your legs and gluteal muscles working. If you wish, clasp your hands behind your back and press them into the floor for extra lift.

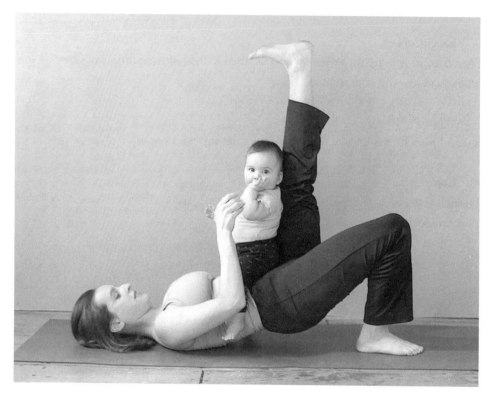

Half Wheel Pose (with Variation)

Baby

Sit your baby on your pelvis as you roll up and down. Then place him on your shins for Flying Child Pose variations.

Essentials

Engage your abdomen and lengthen your tailbone so that you roll through the spine and your back does not arch away from the floor.

What if . . .

If your lower back feels strained, press your feet into the floor, which will help lengthen the back. Do not practice the leg variations.

Cool Thing

This *asana* teaches you how to strongly work your legs without constricting your lower back.

Variation to Strengthen the Legs

- While in Half Wheel Pose, stretch one leg straight up to the ceiling. Your baby can sit on your pelvis leaning against the raised leg. Keep your weight as central as possible and press the standing foot into the floor.
- Take three breaths. Release the pose and repeat with the other leg.

Variation to Strengthen Lower Abdomen

- Start with both legs extended to the ceiling; knees can be slightly bent.
- Create a little seat by placing both hands, palms down, under your sacrum. This action will help support your lower back.
- Slowly lower both legs toward the floor.
- Raise the legs to starting position.
- Repeat 5–10 times.

BABY ENGAGEMENT EXERCISES IN HALF WHEEL POSE

These exercises incorporate an element of peek-a-boo. This is a great way for your baby to learn that you are sometimes close by and sometimes not. As babies begin to make their preferences and abilities known, they may want to use you as gymnastic equipment or only as a checkpoint while they work on their own routines. Both parallel play and tumbling with Mum are great activities. The following exercises add to the Flying Child Pose. They are highly interactive, and most babies love the excitement of them. Plus, they provide additional abdominal and leg-strength work for you.

Flying Child Pose III

Mum

Lie on your back with your knees bent into your chest.

Baby

- Place your baby tummy-down on your shins.
- Bounce your shins (and your baby), occasionally varying the rhythm.
- Bring her in close for kisses by bringing your knees toward your nose.
- With your head up, extend your legs as far away as you can while keeping hold of your baby. Draw your knees back in. Repeat five times.
- Bring your shins (and baby) parallel to the floor and lift your head and shoulders. Holding your baby, raise your feet to the ceiling, letting her slide down your legs onto your chest. She will love to flip to a standing finish. Repeat three times.

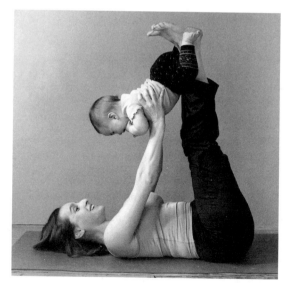 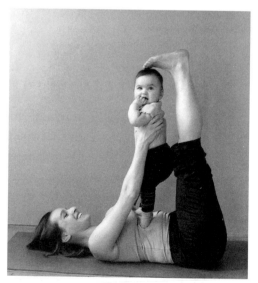

Flying Child Pose III Variation (leg slide)

- With your baby on your shins, roll forward to a sitting position (using your baby's weight to help you). Her feet will probably touch the floor along with yours. Transition into a Seated Forward Bend (*paschimottanasana*) and kiss your baby's stomach.
- Add a Baby Flip! (See page 134).
- Add Baby Presses (if your baby is not too heavy). (See page 115).

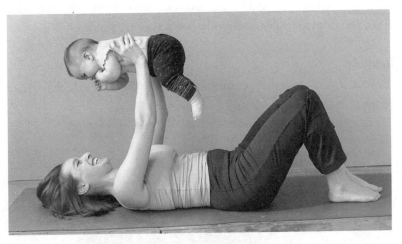

Baby Press

FULL WHEEL (*Urdhva Dhanurasana*)

Mum

- Lie down with your knees bent and slightly apart, your feet on the floor near your pelvis, about hip-width apart.
- Place your hands palm down on the floor near your ears, with your thumbs next to your ears. Your elbows and forearms should be parallel to each other.
- Take a few breaths, and release your shoulders away from your ears.
- On an inhale press your hands and feet into the floor and lift your hips, shoulders, and head off the mat.
- Your waist and pelvis should lift directly from where they are on the mat. Do not let them shift toward your head or your feet.

- Let your head hang relaxed and breathe into the chest.
- To come down, tuck the chin, letting your shoulders touch the mat first, and then slowly roll down the spine onto the mat.
- Take several breaths between back bends. If you are breathing rapidly, wait until the breath returns to normal to do another one.

Baby

Your baby is resting on the floor behind your head so that when you rise up she will see you from a whole new upside-down vantage point.

Essentials

Maintain your legs in a parallel position by relaxing the inner thighs. This will create more space in the lower back and sacral area.

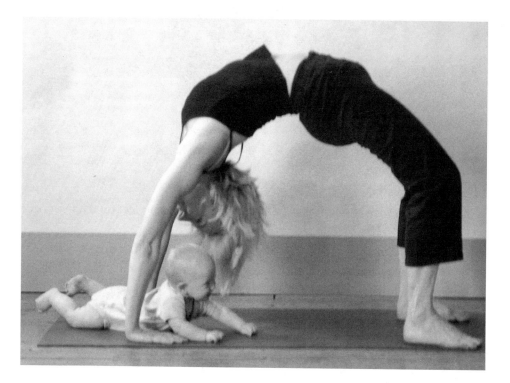

Full Wheel

What if . . .

If you can't press all the way up, work on the Half Wheel version or the variation described below. As your arms get stronger and your shoulders open, this will become easier.

Cool Thing

This pose, like all back bends, opens the chest area. See how alive you'll feel after a few of these.

Variation to Increase Arm Strength

Practice the arm position without putting weight into the arms to increase the range of motion in your shoulders. Then push up and place the top of your head lightly on the floor. This is also a good preliminary step before Full Wheel.

REVOLVED BELLY POSE *(Jathara Parivartanasana)*

With bent legs.

Mum

- Lie on your back with your knees bent into the chest.
- Feel the length of the spine.
- Reach and extend your arms along the floor in line with your shoulders.
- Keep both shoulders on the ground.
- Shift your hips about 5 centimeters to the left so that as you move your legs over to the right, your hips will remain in line with your torso.
- Lower your knees to the right side, hovering a few centimeters off the ground.
- Keep knees together at waist level.
- Keep abdomen and lower back long.
- Stay for a few breaths and use the abdominal muscles to lift your legs to center.
- Repeat on other side.

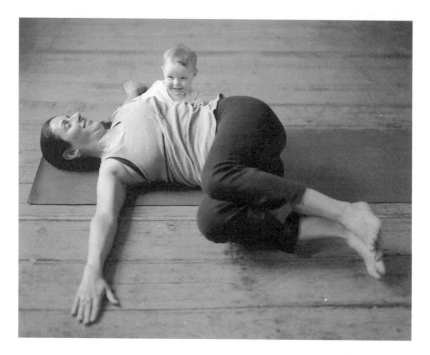

Revolved Belly Pose

Baby

    Your baby can sprawl and crawl all over you. We also suggest lying her along the shoulder opposite your dropped knees, to anchor your shoulder to the mat.

Essentials

Your inner thighs must be together and knees must stay in line.

What if . . .

If you can't get your knees to hover a few centimeters off the ground without straining or shortening your back, lift your knees higher until you can re-lengthen your spine.

Cool Thing

This *asana* really strengthens your abdomen and lower back. It is said to help with digestion and elimination by deeply massaging the intestines.

Straight Leg Variation

Instead of working with bent knees, do the entire *asana* with straight legs.

- Start with legs extended to the ceiling; shift your hips to one side.
- Make sure to keep inner heels tight together.
- Your feet should be 5 centimeters off the floor at shoulder level.
- This pose is much more intensive on the lower torso, so work up to it slowly. Your spine must stay long with the abdomen working strongly before you attempt this variation.

BOUND ANGLE POSE (*Baddha Konasana*)

Mum

- Sit on the mat with the soles of your feet together, as close to the pubic bone as you can get them.
- Lengthen your pubic bone away from your navel and bring your lower back in.
- Keep the outsides of your feet touching and imagine your knees opening away from your hips. This deepens the stretch of your hips and inner thighs, helping to draw your knees away from your body and toward the mat.
- Bend forward over the legs, breastbone toward the mat, while keeping the abdomen and inner thighs relaxed.

Baby

Your baby can sit or stand on your feet, or she can sit in front of you as you lean forward. If locomoting, she can also get behind you and grab hold of your shoulders, going for a ride as you stretch forward.

Essentials

Relax the hip flexor muscles in the front of the hip.

What if . . .

If your knees are really far from the floor, sit on a pillow.

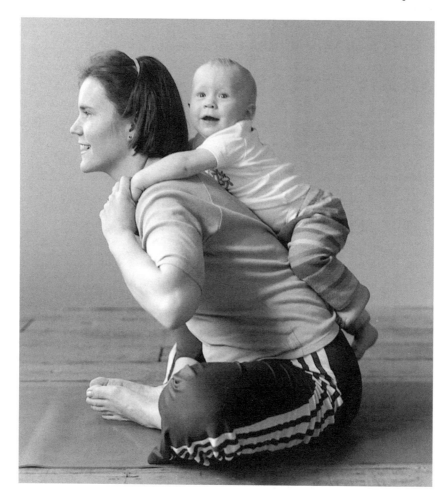

Cool Thing

According to Geeta Iyengar, a major figure in the Iyengar school of yoga, this is one of three essential *asanas* for women. It is a great stretch for the whole pelvic area and is reputed to be beneficial for the reproductive organs.

SEATED FORWARD BEND (*Paschimottanasana*)

Mum

- Sit with your legs extended and together, with knees and toes pointing to the ceiling.
- Lengthen your spine and press backs of your legs into the floor.
- Keep the front of the torso long as you fold forward over your straight legs.
- Aim your lower ribs toward the knees, and the sternum and head toward the feet.
- Keep your collarbones wide and drop your shoulder blades down the back.
- Reach arms toward outsides of feet.

Baby

Your baby is lying across your thighs or on your back as in Bound Angle Pose. She may sit at your feet and catch your hands as you bend forward. Try the baby-rolling exercise below.

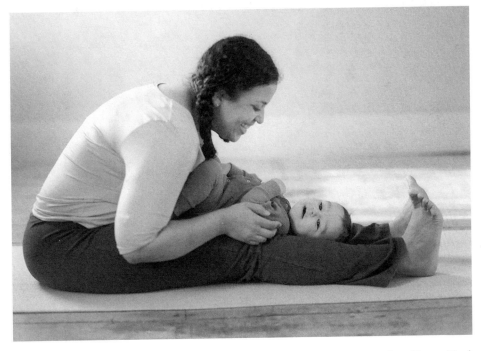

Seated Forward Bend

Essentials

Move forward smoothly with each exhalation; no bouncing. Keep the backs of your legs moving into the floor.

What if . . .

If you feel as if you can't bend forward, or you feel a pull in the back of the knee, sit on a pillow. You can also bend your knees slightly.

Cool Thing

Notice how much more flexible you have become and what a good partner your baby is.

Forward Bend Variation for Baby

• Have your baby sit at the end of your legs, her belly against your feet.
• Hold hands; tickle her belly with your toes.

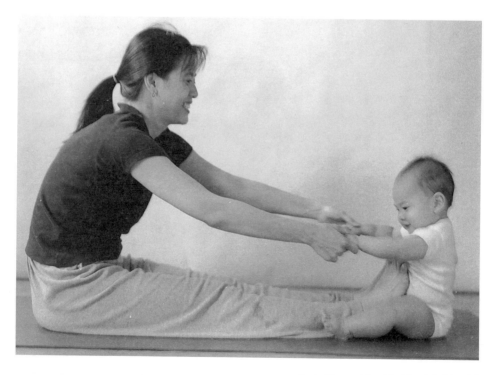

Seated Forward Bend (holding baby's hands)

BABY ENGAGEMENT EXERCISE: BABY ROLLING

Mum

Sit with your legs outstretched and close to each other.

Baby

- Your baby is lying on his stomach across your thighs.
- Gently lift his shoulder and hip closest to you and begin rolling him down the length of your legs.
- Help him place his palms down to push against the mat.
- Roll him back up.

RESTING POSE (*Savasana*)

Mum

- Lie down on your back.
- Completely relax your body.
- Focus on keeping your inhalation and exhalation even.
- Direct your breath through the tips of your nostrils.

Baby

Your baby can nurse or rest with you.

Essentials

Let your weight sink into the ground.

What if . . .

If your back is uncomfortable, put a pillow under your knees or prop your lower legs on a chair.

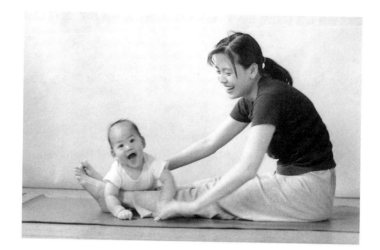

Baby Roll (I)

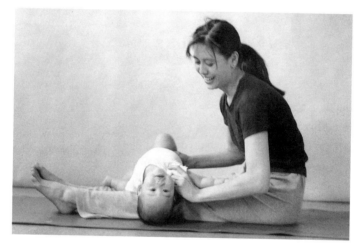

Baby Roll (II)

Cool Thing

Savasana is the great assimilator. If you finish your practice without doing *savasana* your mood may be affected by the last few *asanas* you did. *Savasana* integrates the energy of your entire practice, which will leave you feeling much more balanced and restored.

Savasana Variation for Tight Back

- Place the feet on the floor, comfortably away from hips.
- Let your knees fall inward resting against each other.
- If your baby is not on top of you, drape your arms across your chest so that your hands rest near the opposite shoulder.
- Completely relax.

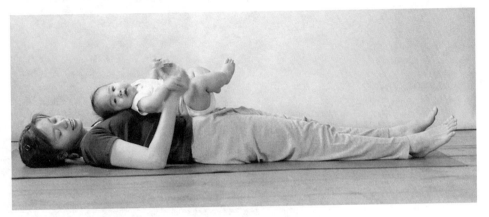

Resting Pose

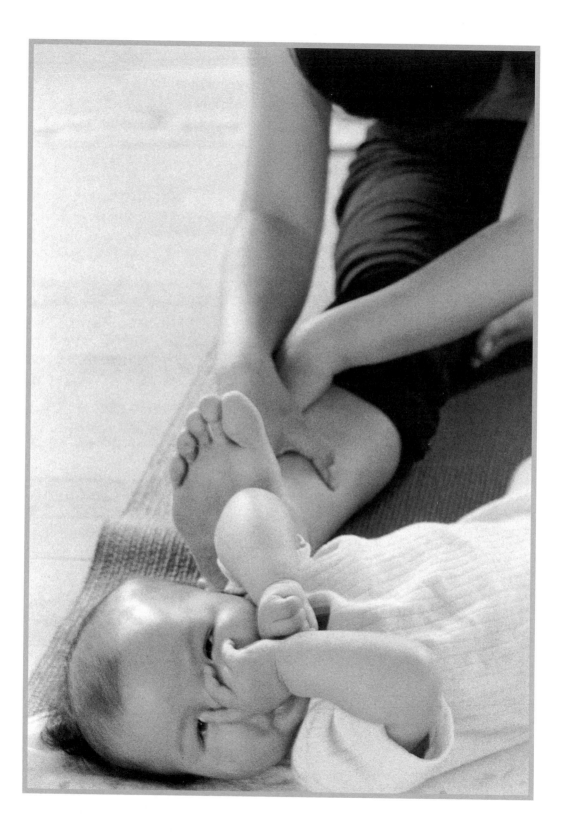

7

CLASS 4:
The Cesarean Section

A RESTORING PRACTICE TO CENTER AND ALIGN
APPROXIMATELY 30 MINUTES; HOLD EACH POSE THREE TO FIVE BREATHS.

Breathing Exercise: Same-Length Breathing

Supine Chest Opener

Half Wheel Pose

Navel Sweeps

Baby Om's Sphinx Variation

Side Tree

Seated Twist

Cat and Cow

Child's Pose

Standing Forward Bend

Wide-Leg Forward Bend

Triangle Pose

Downward Facing Dog

Sage Pose

Legs Up the Wall

As we prepare for childbirth, we never think we'll be the one to have a cesarean delivery. Most of us believe that it will always happen to someone else. Just the term C-section conjures up a sinking feeling and images of knives and white-coated doctors.

When Laura was pregnant, her friend Vicky, mother of a three-year-old, noted that people tend to place too much emphasis on the birth process. This seemed like a mysterious statement at the time, because birth is the major event to which pregnant women look forward. When we're pregnant, we dream of and anticipate our baby's birth; we rehearse the process countless times in prenatal classes and at home. We understand that the process may be strenuous and painful, but we never believe it will end in surgery. In Laura's case, however, she would come to understand how true Vicky's words were. After sixteen hours of labor, Laura, like many women, had a cesarean.

Since yoga is a practice that unites body and mind, it seemed logical that our practice of yoga would prepare us for effective self-management during the birthing process. But while yoga certainly strengthens internal organs and helps focus concentration, the sense of empowerment this imparts must be tempered with the knowledge that childbirth is a process not completely under our control. Sarah's yoga practice certainly helped her manage pain during Rosey's birth. But no level of practice could have predicted or controlled Laura's need for a surgical delivery.

There has been a minor revolution in the politics of childbirth, backed by research indicating that women are holding the reins. Some of the information disseminated to pregnant women is long overdue; some of it is plain silly. For example, Sarah went to a Lamaze class in which women were asked to line up on one side of the room if they wanted drugs during birth and the other side if they didn't. And Laura heard many myths about cesareans, such as the practice of tying a woman's hands down before surgery. The result of misinformation is often fear or an unrealistic sense of responsibility.

Many women participate in prenatal programs that ask them to write out birthing plans with expectations that their bodies will obediently follow the scripts they have imagined. We are encouraged to imagine ourselves as the director, star, and costume designer of our birthing production. If all goes as planned, we receive praise for having a natural childbirth. But if our birthing process diverges from the script—requires pain relief or labor-inducing medications—we end up with sympathy or even disdain. This pressure can make us feel as though having a C-section means we've failed in doing something as "natural" as giving birth. But the idea that it's your fault is one more myth about birth that should be relegated to the trash can of faulty birth lore. We can hardly emphasize this enough: if you have a C-section, remember that it doesn't imply any failure or fault on your part.

Cesareans are now more common than they were in the past, making them a mainstream procedure. "Failure to progress" is the most common reason given by obstetricians for this procedure. After the birth, women sometimes suffer mixed feelings as they question whether or not they or their babies were actually in danger, or if the procedure was really needed. If you ended up having a cesarean for this reason, you may feel cheated because you didn't have a natural birth or angry if you felt the procedure was done unnecessarily. If your life or your child's life was clearly in danger, however, the emotions surrounding a C-section will probably be eased by the sense of relief when the crisis has been averted. According to Lise Eliot, author of *What's Going On in Here?*, the most common serious indications for a cesarean are: abnormal placenta, trapped umbilical cord, baby is too large for the mother's pelvis, or serious illness in the mother. Generally, but not always, cesareans are indicated for breech and multiple births.

If you endured a long labor, an emergency C-section can leave you feeling physically and mentally traumatized. On the other hand, a scheduled C-section may make you feel cut off from the experience of labor and birth. This detachment is a difficult feeling after the extended involvement of pregnancy. These are tough ways to begin motherhood. That is why we emphasize that there is no single "correct" birth process, but many.

If you are one of the millions of women who have had a cesarean, we can tell you through experience that your body will heal, and the delivery of your healthy baby can still be celebrated as a wonderful, fulfilling, and emotionally rich experience. One of our students, Michelle, used to joke about the size of her daughter, Kaitlin, and how she couldn't have been pushed through any birth canal. Her cesarean did not in any way diminish the poignancy of her daughter's first cries.

The Class

Cesareans pose some unique challenges in terms of physical recovery. Surgery is a shock to your body. Your muscles feel weak and tight, and you may feel nervous about undertaking any kind of physical activity. Even carrying your baby may feel like a challenge. We understand this, and have designed the cesarean class to address these challenges. First, and most important, wait at least six weeks to begin, and even then obtain permission from your doctor before starting. Beginning exercise too soon may jeopardize the healing of the incision. Once you're ready to start, however, the first series of *asanas* in Class 4 will gently help your body regain a sense of integrity, openness, and core strength. We avoid lunging, back bends, and wide-leg standing poses because they stretch the abdomen and pelvis, pulling the incision. Even so, look out for your own body: if you feel a tugging sensation when working, stop immediately and return to a place where you no longer feel any pulling.

An added caution: don't move on to Class 2, the 3–6-month class, until you are free of pain around the site of your incision. Class 2 focuses on back bending, which is especially hard on the post-cesarean body. If you still feel pain, your body is telling you to slow down; you should continue to practice the cesarean section class, alternating with class 1 (0–3), and gradually working up to the 3–6-month class. Listen to the needs of your body.

Your Body

These *asanas* will gently help your body regain its flexibility and strength. You will want to work especially slowly so you can rebuild a lasting sense of alignment. With a cesarean birth, you are experiencing all the early postnatal issues as well as dealing with the additional complications of surgery. After several days in a hospital bed and a clear liquid diet, your muscles may feel cramped and sore. Your abdomen will have gotten painfully distended from air in your intestines, and you may be unable to stand up straight for weeks because of the incision across your abdomen. Although your overall recovery from birth will take longer, the good news is that you have suffered fewer traumas to the vagina and pelvic floor than in a vaginal birth.

You may feel that your connection to your body is segmented—that your upper body and lower body are somehow disconnected. Cesarean section is major abdominal surgery, and your body may remember this far better than your mind will. Your midsection will be even weaker than the average postnatal body. You'll need to retrain the abdominals to connect the upper and lower body and support the lower back and abdominal wall. Since your pelvis did not have the experience of pushing out a baby, you won't have to worry so much about overstretched pelvic ligaments. However, you may sense that your pelvic area seems especially tight after surgery, medication, and a longer, slower convalescence. You'll still need to practice your Kegels, to recover from the pressure put on the bladder and urethra during pregnancy.

In addition, the pain around the incision and the effects of medication may depress you. Your anxiety about handling your baby can be increased because of your physical fragility. Any activity you do with your child can help to lessen the intensity of these feelings and may even hasten your recovery.

Lying on your stomach following pregnancy always feels strange and thrilling, but you now have the added discomfort of your incision. Be forewarned, and begin slowly. Wait until your body feels comfortable with this position again. When your abdomen is pressed into the mat as it is in the gentle chest-opening exercises, the pressure on your stomach may begin to feel welcome.

Your Baby

Research has been done on cesarean-birth babies that suggests that these infants do not get some of the important benefits experienced during vaginal birth. Some benefits accrue from maternal hormones released during labor, as well as the squeezing of the uterine contractions and the process of being compressed during passage through the birth canal. Thus we believe there are some simple considerations C-section babies will particularly enjoy. Swaddling is believed to be especially comforting for C-section babies. Laura's son Miles, who was scheduled for cesarean birth because of his breech position, loved to be swaddled. Besides the sucking action, pacifiers are also thought to be comforting because they relax the digestive tract. A C-section baby also benefits greatly from massage. Of course, we're all for massaging babies regardless of how they were born.

The cesarean class was developed to give the mother even more proximity to her baby. The pre-term or cesarean baby may want to be held and comforted for longer periods of time, and much of Class 4 can be done in a soothing manner with your baby on or near your body. If your baby prefers to be swaddled much of the time, don't worry. Infants get a lot of their stimuli visually until about three months of age, so being swaddled in no way makes them feel confined or hinders their physical development. In fact, it may relax them, allowing for more participation, not less!

Note from a Mum

Because I developed a hernia during pregnancy, my choices of exercise are limited. Yoga provides a terrific combination of muscle strengthening and stretching that I can specifically tailor to my needs. I find Baby Om yoga simultaneously relaxing and invigorating. I am not only more energized to care for my active daughter but also feel like I had a good workout. Baby Om yoga also helped me recover from my C-section.

After the birth of my daughter, I felt weak and, in a strange way, disconnected from my own body. Yoga supported a type of body awareness to help me reconnect and realign my mind and body. It also helped me isolate and strengthen particular areas of my body, such as my abdomen and hips, that had been affected by pregnancy and labor. The brief meditation at the end of the practice is an oasis of calmness during my often chaotically busy days.

Baby Om yoga is easy to learn and a pleasure to share with my daughter. My daughter delights in being bounced on my lap during *navasana* and sliding down my legs during Flying Child III. She giggles and squeals during Downward Facing Dog when my hair touches her face. Sometimes I find her imitating my movements or participating by tapping my legs and feet. I can feel her excitement in discovering my body, and through this experience, discovering her own. In addition to this excitement there is also a calmness that develops from our practice. Yoga is a special time for us, reinforcing feelings of closeness and cementing our bond. My favorite part of yoga is when I thank my daughter for sharing the practice. It is this sharing of movement combined with feelings of closeness that make Baby Om unique and invaluable.

—ANDREA, MOTHER OF KATIE

SAME-LENGTH BREATHING

The breathing practice we first recommend for women recovering from a C-section is called Same-Length Breathing or Even Breath. This practice can be done sitting, but we find that when done in the Supine Chest Opener pose described below, the centering effect can be even more powerful. Set up your pose, then completely relax.

- Completely relax your mouth, jaw, and neck area, and keep your hands open, palms heavy, and belly tension-free.
- Inhale through your nose, a long slow breath.
- Exhale through your nose a breath of the same length.
- It helps to count the length of your breath to yourself. For example, each inhale and exhale could last for three counts.

Variation

You can practice directing your inhale toward your back (where it touches the pillows), or anywhere you feel tightness. Use your breath to expand and release each spot.

SUPINE CHEST OPENER

Mum

- Lie back on the pillows so that your upper back is elevated, and your shoulders and hips rest on the ground.
- Release your lower back and buttocks toward your heels.
- Relax the shoulders and soften the back of the neck.
- Extend your legs, first touching, then letting them release away from the center.
- Relax and let your body release slowly, breath by breath.

Baby

Your baby can lie on your chest or beside you on the mat.

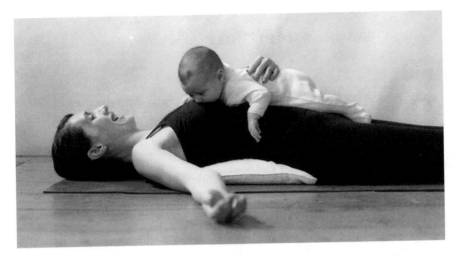

Supine Chest Opener

Essentials

Your chest must be elevated.

What if . . .

If you don't feel your chest opening, add another pillow under your back and support your head with an extra pillow. Let your arms roll out, palms up.

Cool Thing

The longer you can stay in this pose, the better. It helps alleviate fatigue and depression.

Variation

- With your baby next to you on the floor, reach your arms overhead until your knuckles touch the floor behind you.
- Hook your thumbs together and stretch from fingers to toes.
- If you have room, circle your arms out and down.

HALF WHEEL POSE *(Setu Bandhasana)*

Mum

- Lie on your back with your knees bent and your feet on the floor close to the sit bones.
- Inhale, and on the exhale draw your navel strongly toward the floor, engaging your abdominal muscles.
- Keep your knees parallel and press the big toe joints into the mat.
- Keep your collarbones broad and draw your shoulder blades together.
- Press your feet into the mat to lift your hips, and slowly roll up and down along your spine, repeating the movement a few times.
- On the last roll, stay up for several breaths and feel the backs of your legs and gluteal muscles working.

Baby

Sit your baby up and lean her against your thighs or lay her on your chest, where she will ride up and down as you move through the *asana*.

Essentials

Use your abdominal muscles and lengthen your tailbone so that you roll fluidly through the spine. When in the resting position, do not let your back arch away from the floor.

What if . . .

If you feel a strain in your lower back, press your feet into the mat to help lengthen your back, and lift your spine only a few centimeters off the floor. Don't practice the variations until you are more comfortable in this pose. If the baby engagement exercises cause discomfort, don't do them; wait until you gain strength and heal.

Cool Thing

This is a great pose to work on knitting the abdominal muscles toward each other and toning the backs of the legs. Besides strengthening the core of the body, this *asana* massages your back as you roll up and down the spine.

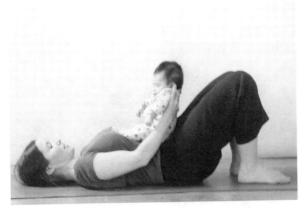

Half Wheel Pose (hips down)

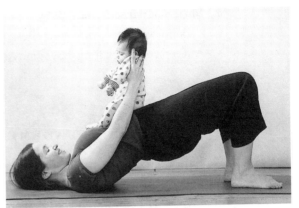

Half Wheel Pose (hips up)

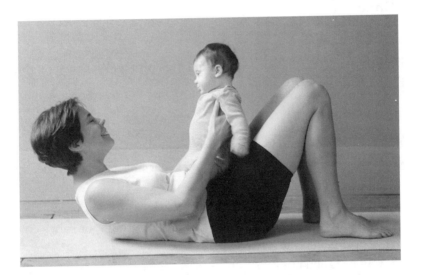

Half Wheel Variation (head up)

Variation to Strengthen the Abdominals

- With your back flat on the floor, exhale, drawing the navel to the spine.
- Lift your head and look at your baby. (Keep the navel drawn in toward the spine.)
- Relax head to the floor. Repeat 5–10 times.

Variation without Your Baby

- Bend your knees into your chest, and slowly lower your feet to the mat.
- Keep your back long, navel moving to the spine. Repeat five times.

BABY ENGAGEMENT IN HALF WHEEL

These exercises are the most basic of our Flying Child poses. This series adds abdominal work to your practice and offers a whole new vantage point from which your baby can watch you. Babies love this active form of play. It is fun for all involved. Feel free to add variations as you see fit.

Flying Child I

Mum

- Begin by lying on your back with your knees bent and your feet on the floor.
- Fold your knees into your chest.

Baby

- Your baby is lying tummy-down on your shins.
- Wrap your hands around her sides with your fingers spread wide, spanning her rib cage.
- Gently bounce your baby by bouncing your shins at a slow pace.
- Gradually increase size and speed of bounces, letting your baby's enjoyment and security guide you.
- Lift your head and bring your knees (and her face) to your nose for a kiss.
- Gently rock your knees side to side (not too far in either direction).
- If you're feeling strong, extend your shins slightly away from you and bring them back in. This will engage your lower abdominals.

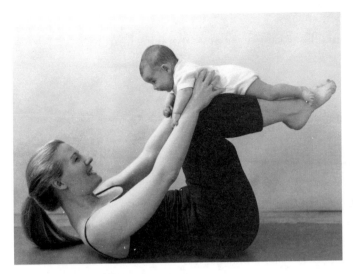
Flying Child (Pose I)

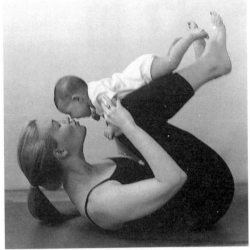
Flying Child Pose (with a kiss)

NAVEL SWEEPS

Mum
- Lie on your back with both knees bent and your feet on the mat.
- Extend the right leg along the ground.
- Draw your navel in toward the spine, engaging the abdominal muscles, and lift the straight right leg to the ceiling.
- Lower the leg (in the longest arc possible) back down to the floor.
- When it reaches the floor, bend the knee and fold it to your chest. Then extend the same leg along the ground and begin again.
- Do not let the back of your hips come off the floor as you sweep the leg to the ceiling.
- Make sure to keep your lower abdomen long and the sacrum touching the floor with the bent leg (this will lift your hips).
- Repeat three to five times.
- Change legs.

Baby

Your baby is either sitting on your chest gazing down at you, or lying heart to heart on your chest.

Essentials

Keep the back long and neck relaxed.

What if . . .

If your back arches off the floor, keep your navel or abdominal muscles drawn inward, and move slowly through the exercise.

Cool Thing

This solid and gentle abdominal exercise is from our dancing days.

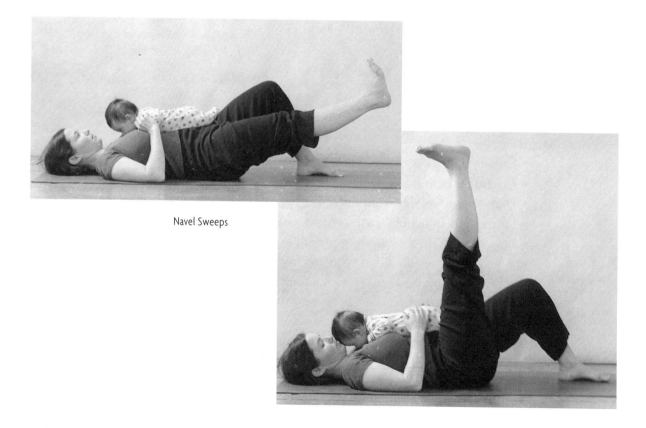

Navel Sweeps

BABY OM'S SPHINX VARIATION

Mum

- Lie belly-down with your elbows and forearms on the ground on either side of your baby with the elbows shoulder-width apart.
- Lift your chest, widen your collarbones, and allow your shoulder blades to drop down your back.
- Keep your head an extension of your spine.

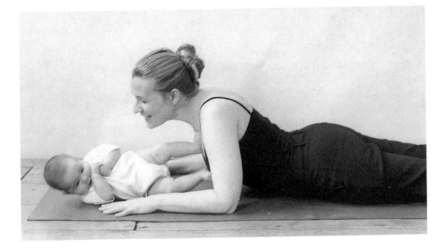

Sphinx Variation (hips down)

Sphinx Variation
(hips up)

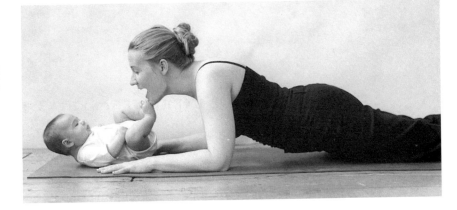

- Slowly begin to lift your hips off the ground (knees stay on the ground) by contracting your lower abdomen muscles back toward your spine. This movement is subtle but strong.
- Keep your back lengthened and your chest opened.
- Release hips down.
- Press your hands into the floor, letting this action lift the breastbone toward the ceiling. The elbows hug the sides of the body.
- Release, breathe, and repeat several times.
- Start by practicing the exercise with your knees on the ground. When that gets easier, try the same exercise with your legs straight. This is much more work for the abdominal muscles, so don't overdo it.

Baby

Your baby is on her back, receiving your gentle squeezes and kisses.

Essentials

Keep pressing the forearms into the ground and lifting your chest up throughout the exercise.

What if . . .

If your lower back feels compressed, think of moving the pubic bone toward the mat.

Cool Thing

This pose opens the chest and works on abdominal strength at the same time.

BABY ENGAGEMENT EXERCISES: SPHINX TUMMY PLAY

During Sphinx Variation, both mother and baby are on their stomachs. If your baby is younger than eight weeks, you may want to prop her up on a cushion that will slightly elevate her torso. The Sphinx Variation may feel very strange to you as well. The memory of your pregnant belly and your instincts to protect it are probably still strong, but it is a great opportunity to model the position for your baby and at the same time strengthen your back and abdomen. During the Sphinx Variation, your baby has the option of resting between your hands, close to your face. It is important for her to have her tummy time as well, so follow your Sphinx practice with these simple exercises and you will soon be doing them in tandem.

Mum
Sit cross-legged.

Baby
Your baby is lying on her belly facing you. You may want to prop up her upper body on a firm flat cushion.

For Baby's Arms
- Try to uncurl your baby's fingers and place each palm on the floor near her shoulders (see illustration on page 28).
- Use a finger-opening stimulus, like rubbing the knuckles together (see illustration on page 27).
- Gently fold in one of your baby's feet toward the opposite buttock, then extend her leg straight. Repeat on the other side.
- Rub the soles of feet together (see illustration, page 29).

Massage
- Give a gentle massage, stroking from your baby's neck to her buttocks, hand over hand.
- Using one finger, stroke the length of her spine from the back of her neck to her tailbone.
- Stroke from the spine out, around the rib cage toward the front ribs.
- Give little squeezes down the backs of her legs followed by long strokes.
- Massage the soles of her feet.

SIDE TREE (*Anantasana*)

Mum

- Lie on your right side with your shoulders, hips, legs, and feet in line.
- Rest your head on your right arm and keep your hips in line, perpendicular to the ground.
- Place the left hand on the floor in front of you for balance.
- Flex your feet as if pressing against a wall.
- Apply *mula bandha* (pelvic floor lift).
- Bring the left foot to the inside of the right inner thigh by bending your knee to the ceiling. (This is tree.)
- Keep the top hip moving down toward the bottom heel. Rotate the upper leg outward and keep the bottom leg very straight.
- The right and left side of the waist should be even.
- Repeat on the other side.

Baby

Your baby is lying on the mat in front of you, maybe nursing.

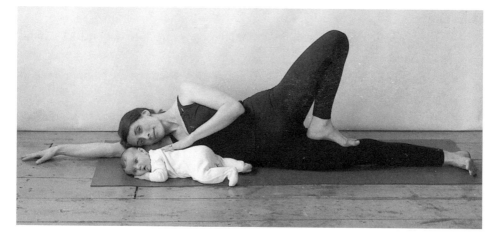

Side Tree

Essentials

Keep the tailbone reaching down toward the extended heel to maintain length in the spine.

What if . . .

If you feel unstable, place your top foot on the floor in front of the extended knee.

Cool Thing

This is a great pose in which to nurse while you reconnect your center without having to work against gravity.

Variation to Stretch Hamstring

- Bend your knee and take hold of your left big toe, ankle, or shin.
- Extend the leg to the ceiling.
- Keep the top hip moving down toward the bottom heel.

Variation with Pillow to Support Back

Place a pillow behind your lower back or hips to keep you from tipping onto your back.

SEATED TWIST (Parsva Siddhasana)

Mum

- Sit cross-legged on the mat, extending down through the sit bones while lengthening the spine and head toward the ceiling.
- Broaden across the collarbones and imagine lifting your heart.
- Place your left hand on the outside of your right knee or ankle, and your right hand on the floor behind you.
- Keep your spine lifted and moving in as you rotate your rib cage around to the right. To support and deepen the twist, use a slight pressure of the left hand into the right knee as the back hand presses into the mat.

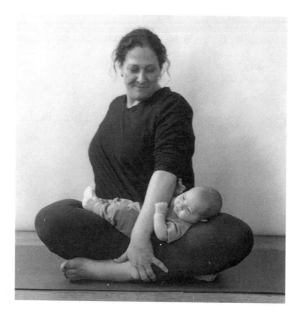

Seated Twist

- Lift your chest and waist as you inhale and deepen the twist as you exhale.
- Relax your neck.
- Repeat on the other side.
- After doing both sides, return to center and sit still.
- Chant *Om* to your baby.
- After you have finished your *Om*(s), practice your Kegels.

Baby

Rest your baby in your lap, sitting or reclining. Smile and gaze at her as you experiment with changing your focus. Play peek-a-boo!

Essentials

Keep the weight even in both sit bones.

What if . . .

If you can't reach the back arm to the mat, move it closer to your body or place your hand on a book.

Cool Thing

What a relief it is to release the back in a twist after not having much mobility in the torso for nine months. This pose is said to relieve congestion in the abdominal cavity.

Variation to Relax the Lower Back

- Sit in a cross-legged position.
- Fold forward over your legs (and baby) and walk your hands forward.
- Keep your sit bones anchored to the mat.
- Walk your hands over to the right until your head and chest are over the right knee. Take a few breaths there.
- Walk your hands back past the center and over to the left and stay for a few breaths.
- Sit up, change the cross of your legs, and repeat.

BABY ENGAGEMENT IN SEATED POSE

These exercises involve your baby in your practice and your baby becomes secure in your attentions. You are warming up your body and your baby is discovering her own through your guidance and touch. Generally we begin with pressure squeezes, then move through your baby's legs, arms, and the whole torso. Experiment, be silly, have fun.

Mum

Sit in a comfortable cross-legged position or gentle wide-leg pose.

Baby

Your baby is lying on her back, feet toward you.

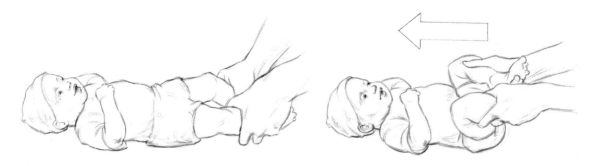

Hands holding baby's legs—legs long

Hands holding baby's legs—knees to chest

Baby Pressure Squeezes

- Squeeze each joint in succession from the center of her body outward (shoulders, elbows, forearms, wrists and hips, knees, ankles). Massage her palms through to each fingertip. (See illustrations on page 27.)
- Massage the soles of her feet through each toe.

For Baby's Lower Body

- Holding your baby's lower legs, press his knees toward his chest and then extend legs as you feel returned pressure. Repeat five times.
- Bicycle his legs in toward his chest one at a time. Repeat five times.
- With both knees to his chest, rock knees from side to side. Repeat five times.
- Place your fingertips under his sacrum or at mid-diaper, and gently bounce him.

For Baby's Upper Body

- Rub the backs of your baby's knuckles together.
- Hold your baby's forearms, slowly crossing them over his chest.
- Gently open his arms to the sides. If you feel resistance give a gentle wiggle and repeat.
- Do this in an easy rhythm: open and close. Keep it simple, but as baby develops, add claps and rhythmic variations such as open and clap, and open and clap, clap.

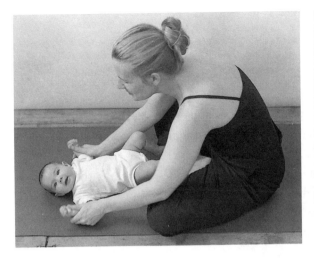

Baby's arms open

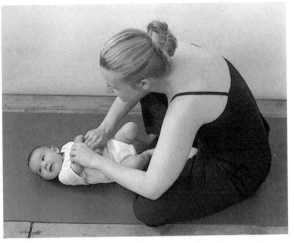

Baby's arms closed

- Circle his arms in both directions.
- Circle his hands around each other (like "the wheels on the bus").

Massage
- Slowly stroke from your baby's shoulders down to his hips.
- Place your thumbs together on your baby's chest and stroke out toward his arms and hands.
- Rub gently from his hips down through his calves, ankles, and feet.
- Stroke his face gently with your thumbs, moving outward from nose to ears.

CAT AND COW

Mum

- Begin on all fours, with your shoulders over your wrists, and your hips over your knees.
- Keep your weight evenly distributed between your hands and knees.
- Draw your navel slightly in toward the spine, lightly engaging the abdominal muscles.
- Spread your fingers apart and put weight into the knuckles as well as the palms of your hands, as if to press the floor away. Your fingers point forward, with the middle fingers of each hand parallel.
- Broaden across your chest, allowing your shoulder blades to move down your back.
- As you inhale slowly, arch your back, bringing the tailbone and head up toward the ceiling (Cow stretch).
- As you exhale slowly, reverse the posture, rounding the back and bringing the tailbone and head down toward the floor, with the navel drawn toward the spine (Cat stretch).
- Repeat three to five times.

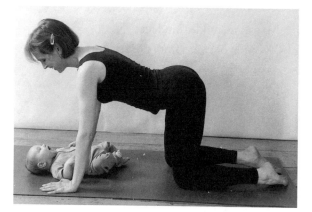

Cow Pose

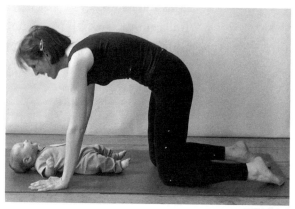

Cat Pose

Baby
> Your baby is lying on the mat with her head directly below your head and chest. She may reach for your face and hair. She is doing what is called pre-reaching, paving the way for her hand-eye coordination.

Essentials
Keep the movement fluid as you do this pose. You are warming up as you glide from Cow to Cat and back.

What if . . .
If you feel a pulling on your incision, focus on the arch in your upper body, making less of an arch in the lower back. If your knees hurt on the floor, place a folded blanket under them for padding.

Cool Thing
You can entertain your baby without having to lift him.

Variation to Release Lower Back
- Start on hands and knees, as in the previous instructions.
- Rock forward, letting your chest move out over your baby and back, your hips toward your heels as in Child's Pose.
- Inhale as you move forward and exhale as you move back. Repeat three times.

CHILD'S POSE (Balasana)

Mum
- Kneel with the tops of your feet on the floor, your toes touching, and your knees apart.
- Bend forward, creasing at your hips. Your hips should remain resting on your heels, with the sit bones pointing down.

- Walk your arms out in front of you to rest your torso comfortably along your upper legs.
- Relax your abdomen and broaden across the lower back.

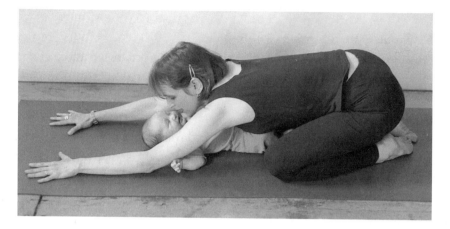

Child's Pose

Baby

Your baby is lying face up on the floor between your knees so you can kiss and cuddle with her as you rest in the pose.

Essentials

This is a restorative pose, so breathe deeply, and release into the pose.

What if . . .

If you can't bring your hips to your heels, place a pillow under your thighs and rest with your elbows on either side of your baby. If you feel as if you're falling forward, give a little pressure backward toward the sit bones, or hug a big pillow.

Cool Thing

This is a great pose for releasing the tension in your belly around the incision. Relax and play peek-a-boo with your baby.

Variation to Stretch Your Feet

- Start by kneeling, with your toes tucked so that you are stretching the "neck" of the toes.
- Keep your inner ankles and calves together. Sit on your heels to deepen the stretch.
- Stay for a few breaths, then release.

Variation to Open Your Chest

- Kneel, with the tops of the feet on the floor, inner feet touching.
- Interlace your fingers, palms touching, behind your back.
- Straighten your arms and roll your shoulders out and back to open your chest.
- Keep diaphragm relaxed and waist long.
- Repeat, changing the interlace of your fingers.

STANDING FORWARD BEND (Uttanasana)

Mum

- Stand with your feet about hip-width apart.
- Bend forward from your hips, keeping your legs straight and kneecaps lifted, engaging the muscles of the thighs.
- Widen and release the lower back.
- Feel the heels pulling to the ground and the sit bones to the ceiling.
- Keep the feet, especially the toes, relaxed and spread.
- Imagine your torso spilling over from the pelvic area like water.
- With every breath, release a little farther toward the mat, dropping your head toward the floor.

Baby

Your baby is lying between your feet on the mat. You can give her a squeeze and rock her side-to-side with the insides of your ankles. As your upper body pours toward the mat, you can easily hold her hands. Look into her eyes and let her gaze draw you forward.

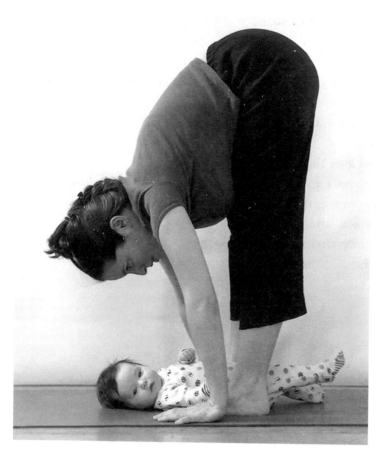

Standing
Forward
Bend

Essentials

Keep the sit bones directly over the heels.

What if . . .

If your hamstrings or lower back feel very tight, let your knees bend slightly.

Cool Thing

This inverted pose is very calming to the nervous system. You can play with your baby while stretching your legs.

Baby Om

Variation to Relax Spine

- From your Forward Bend, bend your knees slightly.
- Round your back and roll up through the spine to standing.
- Your head should be the last to arrive upright.
- Starting with your head, roll down the spine.
- Repeat three times.

Variation for Warming Hamstrings and Back

- From the Forward Bend, inhale and extend your spine, lifting your upper body until it is parallel to the mat. Keep your back flat.
- Draw the navel toward the spine.
- Keep your hips over the heels.
- Hold your baby's hands.
- Exhale and fold back down toward the mat. Repeat.

Restorative Variation

Practice Forward Bend with hips leaning against the wall and feet about 30 centimeters away from the wall. Place a large pillow in your lap and relax the lower back as you extend your spine forward and down.

WIDE-LEG FORWARD BEND (Prasarita Padottanasana)

Mum

- Stand with your feet parallel, about 1.2 meters apart.
- Lift your kneecaps and press the feet into the floor.
- Bend forward to the mat, keeping your spine long.
- Place your fingertips on the ground on either side of your baby.
- Draw the navel toward the spine.
- Lengthen your sit bones to the ceiling and your heels down, keeping your hips directly over the heels.
- Press your inner thighs out and the outer thighs in.
- Broaden across the lower back as you release forward with your head toward your baby.

Baby

Your baby is on the mat between your legs, or slightly in front of you. Cuddle with her and make eye contact as you bend forward.

Essentials

Keep your legs straight, especially stretch the outer knee, and keep the arches of the feet lifted.

What if . . .

If you can't reach the ground, widen your legs or place your hands on a chair or wall.

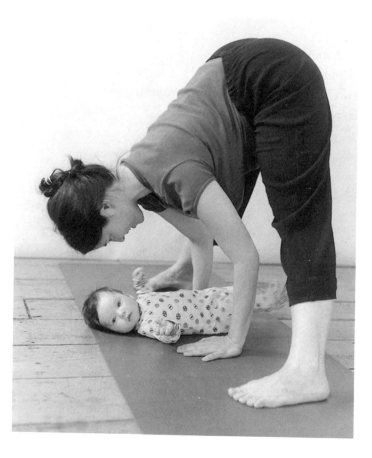

Wide-Leg
Forward
Bend

Cool Thing

In this pose you can get a lot done all at once! It delivers a great stretch for your hips and back, tones the abdomen, calms the mind, and quiets the nervous system. It also has great peek-a-boo potential.

Variation for Spine Stretch

- From the forward bending position, lift your back parallel to the floor, your spine long.
- Walk your hands forward, keeping your hips over your heels.
- Stretch fully from fingertips to sit bones.
- Return to your Forward Bend.

TRIANGLE POSE (*Trikonasana*)

Mum

- Place your feet in a wide stance, about .9 to 1.2 meters apart.
- With your hips facing forward, turn out your right foot 90 degrees and left foot in slightly. The front heel lines up with the arch of the back foot.
- Extend your arms out to your sides, parallel with the floor.
- Straighten your legs and lift the sides of your knees up.
- Lengthen and lift your waist.
- Reach your torso long over the right leg by creasing at the right hip.
- Place your right hand on the shin or ankle for support, and reach your left hand to the ceiling.
- Press the back heel down and extend through the top of the head.
- Open the front of your chest and allow your shoulder blades to slide down your back.
- Keep the abdominal muscles moving in as you take a few long breaths in this pose.
- Repeat on the other side.

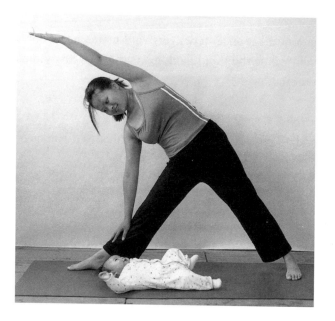

Triangle Pose

Baby

Your baby is lying by your front foot. (When you change sides, turn around so that the other foot is next to your baby).

Essentials

Keep the sides of your waist reaching evenly. Imagine you are moving between two walls.

What if . . .

If you feel a pull on your incision, omit the arm circles and lift your torso up to reduce the stretch. You may also narrow the width of your stance.

Cool Thing

Here is a mainstay standing pose you can practice with minimal or no pull on your incision, and it may be one of the first poses your child imitates. Triangle Pose is a fantastic stretch for the whole body, especially your hips and spine.

Arm Variation to Open Chest

Bend the top arm at the elbow and place it behind your back with the palm facing out. Spiral your chest toward the ceiling and keep reaching the fingers of the bent arm toward the inner thigh of your front leg.

Arm Circle Variation

Circle the top arm over your head and past your baby, tickling him as you pass by. He will learn to anticipate each approaching arm circle.

DOWNWARD FACING DOG *(Adho Mukha Svanasana)*

Mum

- Start in Cat and Cow neutral position, neither arched nor rounded (see page 194).
- With your fingers spread wide, distribute the weight evenly throughout your hands.
- Tuck your toes under and float your hips up and back toward the ceiling (feet are almost mat-width apart).

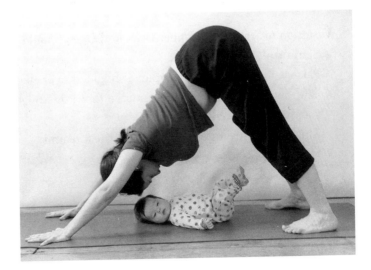

Downward Facing Dog

- Straighten your legs, move your thighs back, and lift the kneecaps.
- Reach down with your heels and stretch your toes forward.
- Press and lengthen, from the hands to the sit bones, making one long line.
- Draw the lower abdomen in toward the spine.
- Release your head and neck, letting your head drop slightly toward your baby.

Baby

Your baby is lying on the mat directly below your chest, resting so that you meet eye to eye when in the pose. Say hello as you move into the position.

Essentials

Extend your spine into one long line, thinking of the sit bones as the high point of the pose. Draw the navel in and up as you lift your abdomen and lengthen the sides of the waist.

What if . . .

If your lower back hurts or if your back is very rounded, bend your knees slightly and try again to extend the spine, moving your hips up and back.

Cool Thing

Think of your pelvis floating toward the ceiling. This can make the pose feel lighter.

Variation to Strengthen Upper Body and Open Shoulders

- Start on all fours.
- Place your forearms on the ground, shoulders over elbows.
- Without letting your shoulders move forward, straighten your legs and lift your hips to the ceiling.
- This is a Downward Facing Dog from the forearms.
- Hold this pose for a few breaths.

SAGE POSE *(Bharadvajasana I)*

Mum

- Start by sitting on your heels.
- Shift your hips to the right until the left hip rests securely on the mat.
- Use your right hand against the left thigh to rotate your torso to the left.
- Keep the right hip moving down away from your waist and lift your chest up and around to the left.
- Broaden the collarbones.
- Think of twisting around a central axis.
- Hold for several breaths, then unwind and twist in the opposite direction.
- Repeat on other side.

Baby

- Your baby is sitting on your lap, supported by your right arm as you twist to the right.

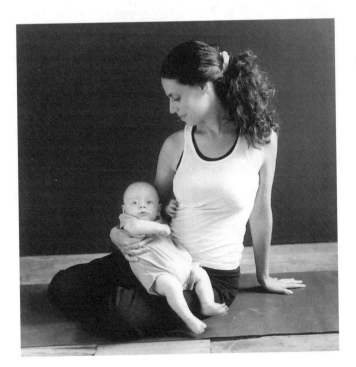

Sage Pose

- Turn your head to gaze back at him, creating a double twist.
- Use your hand to keep him safely on your lap.

Essentials
Keep the back hip weighted down and your spine long.

What if . . .
If you feel any pull on your incision twist less or practice Child's Pose. If you feel discomfort in your lower back, relax the twist in your hips and work on the rotation in the upper body.

Cool Thing
You can twist the upper body without stressing your incision. This is a great release for the spine without being too strong a twist. Also, you can do it while nursing.

LEGS UP THE WALL (*Savasana*)

Mum
- Lie on the floor with your buttocks up against the wall, as if you are sitting on the wall.
- Lengthen your legs up the wall and let them part slightly.
- Release everything: abdomen, thighs, pelvis, rib cage, chest, neck, and head.
- Let your legs roll out as you deeply relax.
- Stay in the pose for as long as you can—five to ten minutes is ideal.
- You can also place a cushion under your hips.

Baby
Your baby relaxes here, too, chest to chest or resting against your thighs.

Essentials
Soften your abdomen.

What if . . .

If your lower back is lifting off the floor, move hips away from the wall. Your back and legs should be comfortable.

Cool Thing

You can actually feel excess fluid leaving your legs. They'll feel cooler and lighter when you are finished.

Variation

- Place the soles of your feet together with knees open into Bound Angle Pose (see page 164) up the wall, or fold your legs into a cross-legged position.
- Stay for a few breaths then switch your crossed legs.

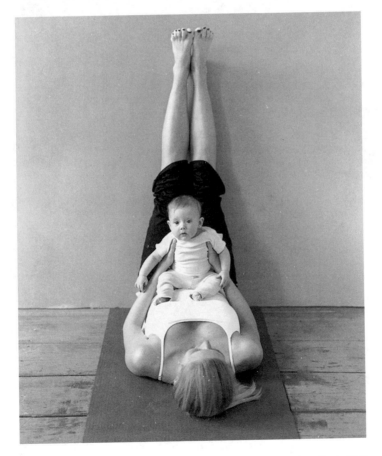

Legs Up the Wall

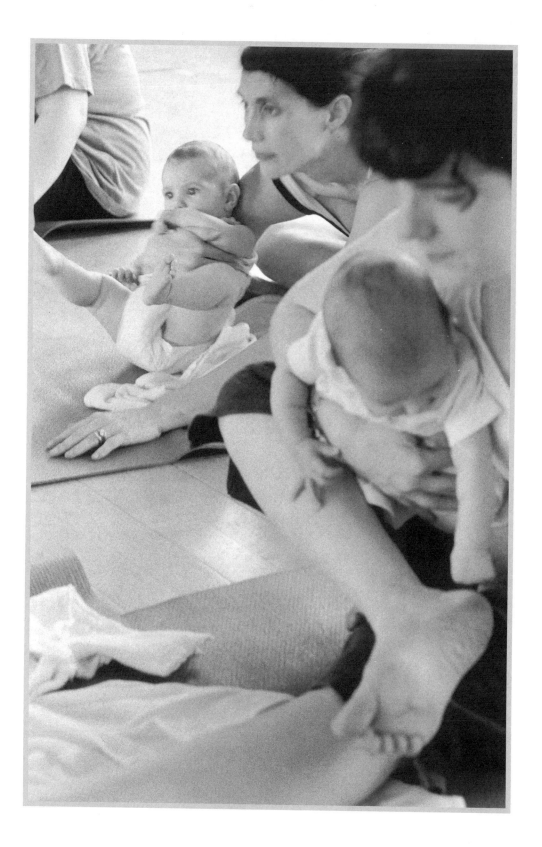

8

Yoga for Nursing and Colic

Yoga for Nursing

Feeding and comforting your baby are part of the big picture of parenting; the one you will probably find yourself engaged in most often is either nursing or bottle feeding. So we have compiled a group of poses that can be done while nursing. You'll find these to be peaceful, seated poses. Many can be done with your back supported by a wall or sitting on a cushion, which will take the strain out of your back. The majority of these *asanas* will stretch your hips and lower back so experiment with ways to make them fun and comfortable. They can be a welcome change from the couch. Make sure you have at least one extra cushion available as an armrest. Each pose may be modified according to your body and your baby's preferences.

Sitting Pose
- Sit with your back against the wall.
- Cross your legs.
- Place your baby in your lap.

- Close your eyes to help you relax and breathe deeply.
- Change the cross of your legs periodically.

Cow Facing Pose

- Sit on the mat with your right leg crossed over your bent left leg, knee over knee, or keep your bottom leg straight if your hips feel too tight (modified Cow Facing Pose).
- Your top leg will support your baby like a pillow.
- Change sides.

Ankle to Knee Pose

- Sit on the mat and bend your left leg.
- Bend your right leg and place right ankle across left knee.
- Line up your shins, if possible.
- Rest your baby on your top thigh, close to the hip.
- Keep both sit bones evenly on the floor.
- Lean slightly forward to open hips and change legs periodically.
- If the top knee is very far from the bottom leg, don't do this pose—do modified Cow Facing Pose instead.

Bound Angle Pose

- Sit with your back against the wall.
- Place the soles of your feet together.
- Place your baby on a cushion on your lap.
- Lean slightly forward (optional).
- Breathe into the stretch.

Sage Pose

- Kneel with your hips off to the right, resting on the mat.
- Your baby will lie in your lap or on a cushion to lift her toward you.
- Twist to the right, using your left hand to support your baby.
- Change sides.

Side Tree

- Lie on your right side with your legs extended.
- Your baby can nurse in the side-lying position.

- Bend your left knee and place your foot on the inside of your right thigh.
- For balance, place your left hand on the floor on the far side of your baby.
- Work on the rotation of your bent leg, keeping hips stacked perpendicularly to the floor.
- Change sides when you change breasts.

Resting Pose
- Lie on your side or your back.
- Nurse as is comfortable.
- Close your eyes, slow your breath, and let the weight of your body release into the floor.

Yoga for Colic

Colic is a big mystery. An accurate definition still eludes us, but typically babies who are colicky have crying jags and are more difficult to soothe and less equipped to "self-soothe." Intestinal distress, which can include excessive gas, heartburn, and reflux, is thought to be a major source of colic. It can be heart-wrenching, maddening. Mostly colic and/or fussiness worsens in late afternoon and at night.

As a result of our own parenting and teaching experiences, we encourage mums of fussy babies to try to work around the fussy times by practicing in the morning or an hour after feeding, when your baby is well rested. Of course, you won't insist on finishing your practice if your baby is inconsolable. You always have the option of putting your Baby Om practice temporarily on hold until your baby is more receptive. Eventually, he will grow out of this condition. We have had some success at soothing, or at least distracting, a fussy baby in our classes. Fussy babies generally like to be held, a phenomenon we have seen over and over. We once gave an entire class of seated poses, so the mothers could hold their babies.

One thing about colic we've learned is that some babies respond positively to a lot of surrounding stimuli while others respond to exactly the opposite. Sometimes the same *asana* is indicated for both temperaments, because it is the quality and intention with which you do something that creates the mood. The same pose or activity can be done in an exciting or a soothing way. First, notice what consoles your baby when he's upset. Is it jiggling, walking, and riding around (enjoying stimuli), or is it a dark room, a hushed voice, and swaddling (enjoying serenity)? In terms of your yoga practice, notice what your baby responds to. The following are two short sequences of *asanas* that may relieve both you and your baby.

Yoga and Your Stimuli-Loving Baby

Rosey was a perfect example of the stimuli-seeking baby when distressed. She hated being swaddled, threw her arms out of the blanket, and refused to be constrained. She loved the Leopard Swing, her little body draped on one of her parent's forearms, one hand coming up supporting her from below, the other hand from above. A successful stimuli-loving technique has lots of motion.

Sun Salute
- Start on all fours, your baby between your hands on the floor (use your exhale to tickle her with your breath).
- Inhale into Cow, exhale into Cat.
- Inhale into Cow, then exhale into Downward Facing Dog.
- Inhale into Plank.
- Exhale into Downward Facing Dog, inhale your knees to the ground.
- Exhale back into Child's Pose.
- Remember to make lots of eye contact while moving through the poses, giving plenty of kisses when in Child's Pose.

Warrior II
- Start with your feet about 1.2 meters apart.
- Sit your baby facing out on your front thigh, using your hands around her waist and chest to support her.
- Slowly bend and straighten your front leg, giving your baby a little ride as you work in and out of the pose.

Baby Arcs
- Stand with your legs comfortably apart.
- Place your baby along your forearm, as in the Leopard's hold.
- Use your second hand to securely support his chest and head.

- Swing him away and toward you. If you have a mirror, swing toward it for added fun and distraction.

Half Wheel Spine Rolls
- Lie on your back, knees bent and feet on the floor.
- Place your baby on your lower abdomen.
- Roll up and down through the spine, adding a gentle bounce of your sacrum. Babies like this little horsey type of ride.

Flying Child Pose
- Lie on your back with your knees bent in to your chest.
- Your baby is draped stomach down on your shins, her head just peeking over your knees. Hold her around her rib cage.
- Bounce your baby and shins, varying the timing and rhythm of the bounces.
- Lift your head and give a gentle puff of air as you rise up for a kiss.

Flying Baby Presses
- From the Flying Child Pose, bring your baby to your chest, your hands still spanning his rib cage.
- Press him directly up over your chest, then bring him down, welcoming him with kisses.
- After repeating a few times, lift him high and sway him gently side to side.

Modified Boat Pose
- Sit with your knees bent, together in front of you.
- Place your baby facing away from you on your thighs; her chin will just reach over the edge of your knees.
- Stroke her back with a hand-over-hand massage.

Seated Forward Bend
- From the Modified Boat Pose, straighten your legs.
- Place your baby either on or between your legs face up.
- Or place him tummy down across your upper thighs.
- Bend forward and soothe him with the sound of your voice and the closeness of your body.

WHEN YOUR BABY NEEDS ACTIVE COMFORT

Laura is a big believer in swaddling and Miles loved it. Even at five months of age it still calmed him. When Miles got irritable, something that really helped was direct, calm, soothing eye and verbal contact. When your baby needs a lot of active comfort, try to keep your energy level as calm as possible and get down on the mat right on his level. Really see eye to eye if you can.

Child's Pose

- Sit on your heels, feet together, knees apart.
- Place your baby between your knees.
- Fold forward and create a soothing, warm place for your baby.
- Stay for a while, releasing your back.

Downward Facing Dog

- Start on all fours.
- Your baby is on the mat below your heart.
- Lift your hips and straighten your legs into Downward Facing Dog.
- Come face-to-face with your baby.

Standing Forward Bend

- Stand with your feet hip-width or wider apart.
- Your baby is between your feet.
- Bend forward and rub his stomach as you gaze into his eyes.
- Try doing small circles with his arms.

Wide-Leg Forward Bend

- Stand with your feet parallel and about 1.2 meters apart.
- Bend forward and bring your fingertips to the floor on either side of your baby.
- Make eye contact with your baby.
- Try walking your hands out forward past your baby.

Modified Boat Pose

- Sit with your knees bent, together in front of you.
- Place your baby facing in toward you.
- Give a gentle hand-over-hand massage along his abdomen.

Seated Forward Bend

- From Modified Boat Pose, straighten your legs.
- Place your baby either on or between your legs, facing you.
- Bend forward and soothe her with the sound of your voice and the closeness of your body.

Resting Pose

- Place your legs on a chair and your baby on your chest as you rest.

OTHER COLIC SUGGESTIONS

- Place your baby high on your shoulder. The pressure may soothe a distressed stomach.
- Swaddle and place your baby facedown (to help relieve gas). Rub her back, head, and forehead.
- Pump one or both of her legs to help relieve gas.
- Give her a warm bath and a massage with baby oil or lotion.
- Play your favorite music and dance, swaying to the music.
- Change your location.
- Put your baby in a carrier and take a walk.
- Try taking your baby for a ride in the car or a trip on the subway.
- Encourage pacifier use as sucking relaxes the digestive tract.
- Try aromatherapy: place some lavender oil on a cotton ball and pass the soaked cotton ball under the baby's nose.
- It may be that nothing you do will relieve your baby's colic, so it's important to try and stay relaxed. Breathe and remember that this will pass.

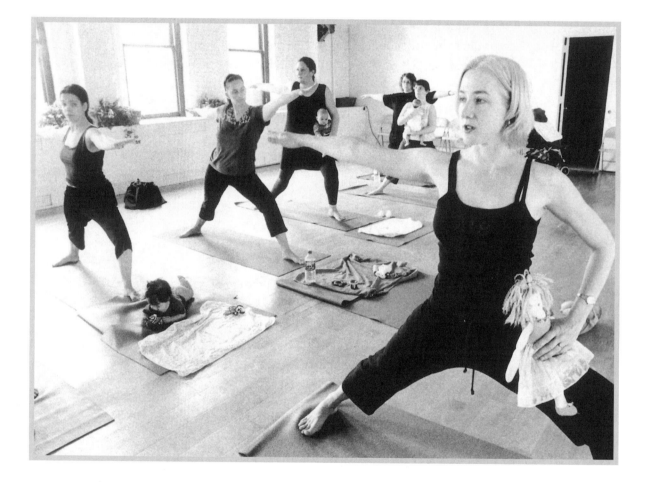

9
Yoga and Postpartum Depression

Written with Johanna Simpson, M.S.W.

The myriad images snapped following a child's birth are supposed to show an elated mother, a beaming father, and a sleeping or crying infant. However, there are other unphotographed images surrounding birth that are swept under the rug, rarely discussed, images that seem to be a question of shame and embarrassment. The new mother who can't bond with her child, cries constantly, can't do things as simple as wash her hair, or walk out the door—she's invisible. Everything seems futile to her. Hopeless, she feels unworthy of her baby and everyone around her. The best anyone can say is: *You're supposed to be happy. Snap out of it, please.* These are some of the hidden images of postpartum depression, a condition in which waves of hopelessness bring a new mother's life to a standstill. Family members and friends tell her to just stop it, as if emotional switches could be turned off and on from some mental power plant.

We've included this chapter on depression for much the same reasons that we included a medical chapter—because we believe women need it. From the stages of labor to the purchasing pros and cons of cribs and diapers, it seems as if every aspect of a baby's entry into the world is discussed. That is, all except the new mother's depression, which still exists as taboo.

If you're affected by postpartum depression you'll feel overwhelmed on a much larger scale than the routine way new parents are overwhelmed by the changes a new baby brings. Feelings of hopelessness and despair, and crying for no obvious reason are all symptoms that come on the heels of exhaustion. Sleep deprivation can make you forgetful and unable to form complete, intelligible sentences. A new baby is terra incognita for most of us, and birth brings with it the extreme and contradictory emotions of love and fear. When new physical and emotional demands leave no time to accomplish even simple things like making a cup of coffee, one is easily pushed over the edge.

Postpartum depression is a force to be reckoned with, as those who have experienced it will tell you. It not only affects the new mother but also interferes with mother-child bonding. Overwhelming feelings of despair can be so powerful that they interfere with the day-to-day demands, both physical and emotional, of parenting. Much has been written about the relationship of exercise and depression. One of the proven ways to help depression (nonmedically or therapeutically) is with exercise. In treating depression, women who don't want to take medication or who are breast-feeding may find some relief through yoga. Yoga class provides exercise, physical contact, and interaction with babies that will ease symptoms and in turn help the bonding/attachment process. It isn't a magic wand to make you and your baby calm and serene. It doesn't clean the house or change diapers, but by training the body and mind to focus and work together, you may find tranquillity and keep anxiety at bay.

Bear in mind that you're not alone. Postpartum depression, a hidden, rarely discussed condition, is as much a part of the post-birth experience as being awakened in the middle of the night. It has many causes and few ways in which it can be alleviated. Women should never be blamed for depression. Its causes are complicated, ambiguous, and the resulting effects of this condition, whether chronic or temporary, are far-reaching. Professional help is an important option and should certainly be sought.

Am I at Risk?

No one knows for certain what causes postpartum depression. It is widely believed that the powerful combination of natural hormone fluctuation, psychological and emotional stress, fatigue, and the overwhelming change in lifestyle that occurs after childbirth creates fertile ground for the formation of depressive symptoms. It is commonplace for women to experience emotional ups and downs after childbirth. The term "baby blues" was coined to explain why so many mothers feel down or blue within the first few days or weeks after giving birth.

However, it is important to make the distinction between feeling blue for a short period of time after childbirth and experiencing stronger feelings of depression that last a much longer time. Typical symptoms associated with the baby blues can be a sad or irritable mood, loss of energy, a feeling of worthlessness or hopelessness, and spontaneous crying. These symptoms typically last from a few days to two weeks. Women who suffer from postpartum depression experience similar symptoms. But for them the symptoms are more severe and can last from two weeks to over a year.

Certain characteristics make postpartum depression somewhat more likely. Women have an elevated probability of experiencing postpartum depression if they (1) have had prior episodes of depression; (2) have a family history of postpartum depression; (3) have a lower level of emotional support from those around them; or

(4) have experienced similar symptoms after a previous birth. These are only weak predictors, however. Some women with a likely history for having postpartum depression never get it and some women who have no obvious risk factors do. This is why it is extremely important to be aware of the signs and symptoms of postpartum depression.

Does It Put My Baby at Risk?

It is well established that the formation of a bond between a mother and her baby is critical to the mental and physical health of the baby. Events that disrupt the process of bonding can have negative consequences. Postpartum depression is one of the disruptions that can, if untreated, have severe negative consequences for both the mother and her child. If untreated, it can seriously interfere with a mother's ability to care for her own and her baby's needs. On the other hand, postpartum depression is highly treatable and women often respond well and quickly to several different treatment options.

Signs and Symptoms

It is important to recognize that postpartum depression is a medical illness and not reflective of the quality of the mother. Too often, women who suffer from postpartum depression also experience extreme guilt and shame about not being happy with the baby, not bonding with the baby, or wishing that the baby had never been born. In our culture, there is an incredible amount of pressure and expectation for new mothers to "glow," and feel that a baby is the best thing that ever happened to them. Women who suffer from postpartum depression, through absolutely no fault of their own, are unable to feel these things. The guilt and shame they consequently feel lead many women not to seek treatment and often not to tell anyone about their symptoms.

Like any illness, postpartum depression can range quite dramatically in severity. Women who are diagnosed with a mild case of postpartum depression may experience the following symptoms for a prolonged period of time: sad mood, low energy, low self-esteem, poor concentration, and a feeling of hopelessness. These symptoms can be accompanied by a feeling of dread about attending to their baby's needs, spontaneous crying spells, and sometimes wishing the baby had never been born.

Symptoms of postpartum depression move along a continuum until they reach the level of severe postpartum depression. Symptoms of severe postpartum depression mirror those of depression: a sad mood for most of the day nearly every day, loss of interest or pleasure in almost all activities, significant weight gain or loss, sleep disturbances, a feeling of worthlessness or excessive and inappropriate guilt, and a diminished ability to think and concentrate. These symptoms can last over two weeks and occupy most of a mother's waking day. They can also be accompanied by feeling like a "bad" person, with recurrent thoughts of death or suicide.

At the most dangerous end of this continuum are repeated thoughts of hurting or killing yourself or your baby, planning how to do it, or starting to hear voices that others cannot hear (hallucinations). If you are experiencing any of these symptoms, you need to seek professional help immediately. Again, we want to stress that you are not at fault. These are physical and psychological symptoms that are beyond your immediate control but can be treated.

How Untreated Postpartum Depression Can Affect Babies

When a mother is depressed there are two forces simultaneously at work that create a negative impact on her baby. First, postpartum depression affects women physically as well as emotionally. Depression can alter your patterns of sleep and eating, and your ability to regulate your own mood and affect. Depressed mothers tend to show less physical affection, provide less visual and verbal stimulation, and engage their babies in play less than nondepressed mothers. When a mother is depressed, her facial expression and tone of voice can become flat and limited in range.

Second, during the same time period that mothers are most likely to experience symptoms of postpartum depression, babies are in a stage of critical development. From one to six months of age, babies are learning how to relate to the world directly from their interactions with caregivers. These interactions, mainly through facial expressions and tone of voice, are how babies learn to attach to caregivers, smile socially, respond to parents' playful behavior, and regulate their own affect.

Babies learn their own range of affect by mirroring that of their caregivers. When a mother is depressed and unintentionally shows her baby primarily negative facial expressions or no facial expression at all, the child learns to imitate the same flat affect and lower activity level. A mother who is suffering from postpartum depression may unintentionally express less affection and be less attentive to her baby's needs. Some long-term effects in babies of untreated postpartum depression can range from depressed facial expressions to increased levels of irritability, short attention span, and sleep and feeding problems—the same symptoms that affect mothers.

It is important to keep in mind that the long-term negative effects on babies occur when they receive prolonged periods of inattention from a depressed caregiver. Feeling sad and tearful for a few months is not going to have a negative effect on your baby. However, as the severity and the time increase, the effects begin to worsen.

Treatment Options
for Postpartum Depression

Treated promptly, the effects of postpartum depression can be kept to a minimum. But treatment depends on proper diagnosis, which is often hampered by the symptoms of the condition itself. Women suffering from depression are often consumed by feelings of guilt and shame. That, coupled with the loss of physical and emotional energy, makes them reluctant, if not downright unable, to seek help.

The first step in helping yourself is educating yourself about the signs and symptoms of postpartum depression and the available treatment options. The most important thing you can do for yourself and your baby is to seek professional help. Mental health professionals are trained to diagnose and treat postpartum depression. Postpartum depression is often treated with medication or therapy and generally a combination of both is considered the most effective. Just as symptoms vary according to the severity of the depression, so do the treatments. Psychotherapy is always a good treatment option. Talking to someone about your fears and guilt can be helpful. A psychotherapist will help you understand your feelings and come up with positive strategies for helping you improve and treat your depression. Medication is sometimes, but not always, an important component of treatment. Some women prefer not to take antidepressant medication or any medications for a variety of reasons, including the fact that many antidepressants are transmitted through breast milk. Express all such concerns to your health care provider and weigh all the risks and benefits to your own situation.

Once you have begun an appropriate course of treatment, adding yoga practice can increase its benefits and help relieve some of your symptoms. It has long been known that exercise releases endorphins in your brain that work to improve mood and energy levels. While the idea of running or aerobics classes may seem far too ambitious in your present state, yoga releases the same positive endorphins as other forms of exercise and has the same effect of improving mood and energy levels.

What makes Baby Om particularly effective is that when you do yoga with your baby you are increasing the physical and emotional connections between you. If your depression symptoms make it difficult to spend hours cooing and smiling at your baby, doing yoga exercises with her can provide an opportunity for bonding. The physical touch and one-on-one connection with your baby during yoga exercises can strengthen the connection you both have for each other.

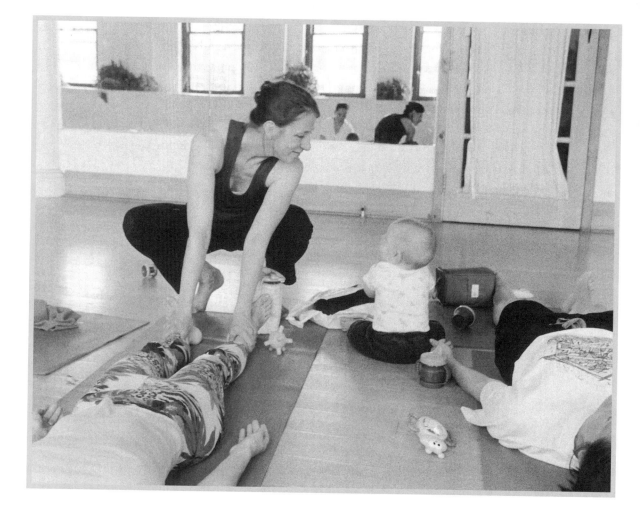

10

The Birth Process and
Its Physical Impact

WRITTEN WITH JENNIFER STATON,
M.S., N.P., R.N.

Y ou may ask what's all this medical stuff about the placenta and the stages of
labor doing in *Baby Om*? Well, we wanted to include some technical information that would be useful in the course of recovery and some technical
definitions that illuminate where our bodies have been and where they're going.
Pregnancy is a window into your body. We get to learn how things work. Body parts
you took for granted or never thought about twice suddenly have shifted their function or behave differently. Where is my pelvic floor? What is a real contraction? For
some women the experience of pregnancy is, thankfully, their only brush with the
medical world, but we do suddenly enter the land of mysterious terminology.

We can talk about physical activity in terms of bending and stretching, but
we thought it would be helpful to know a little more about the pelvic floor and
what's going on there as well as other functional information. Think of this chapter
as a glossary. Some of this information may not be pertinent to your interests or
conditions; other parts you may turn to avidly. Whether you approach this chapter

with mild or eager curiosity, it is meant to clarify physical events surrounding pregnancy in greater detail.

Having undergone very different birth experiences ourselves, and having created Baby Om partially in response to those experiences, we felt it would be interesting to include a brief description of the processes of labor and childbirth in this book. Being inquisitive, we wanted all the gory details! What follows includes medical terminology that may initially be confusing, but most terms are defined in simple English when first presented. Additionally, having noted that postpartum urinary incontinence is a common complaint among our students, we felt it was important to include a section addressing the performance of Kegel exercises, which integrates naturally into the practice of yoga. Engaging the *mula bandha*, or root lock, utilizes the same musculature as Kegel exercises.

Note from a Mum

Baby Om reintroduced me to my body. I'd forgotten what it was like not to be pregnant. Yoga with Sam enabled me to get back my body while still remaining attached to my new baby. I was also happy to be surrounded by other mothers—many first-timers like me. I had a lot of questions and the class was the perfect place to ask them. I felt completely comfortable to be at whatever level I chose. I could push myself, lie down (or fall down!), or nurse. There was support but never pressure. And there was much-needed humor but always within a solid structure.

—NITZA, MOTHER OF SAM

Vaginal Birth

The process of childbirth actually begins several weeks before the onset of "true" labor. Maternal estrogen levels peak weeks beforehand, perhaps in reaction to fetal production of adrenal stress hormones, causing the uterine muscle (myometrium) to be more sensitive to oxytocin and less responsive to progesterone. Oxytocin is a hormone produced by the pituitary gland of the mother, and in smaller amounts by the fetus, which causes uterine contractions. Progesterone is a hormone produced by the placenta in large quantities during pregnancy and acts to quiet the myometrium, preventing unwanted contractions. Braxton-Hicks contractions are the result of these early hormonal changes and are often classified as "false" labor. Eventually, fetal production of oxytocin and placental release of prostaglandins (chemical irritants that stimulate uterine contraction) cause increased maternal production of oxytocin, and the contractions of true labor begin. Labor technically consists of four stages, although the final two stages occur after delivery of the baby.

The first stage of labor begins with the onset of "true" contractions and ends when the cervix is fully dilated (opened) and effaced (thinned and flattened). Labor contractions begin at the top of the uterus, gradually moving downward toward the vagina as this stage of labor progresses. A combination of downward pressure from the fetal head and the progressive downward contractions of the uterus cause the cervix to soften, thin, and pull up into the body of the uterus. Toward the end of this process, the mucus plug is dislodged from the cervix and the mother may notice a small amount of blood-tinged mucus from the vagina (bloody show). The fetal head, which had been floating in amniotic fluid above the pelvis, descends into the maternal pelvic inlet, a maneuver called engagement. Engagement of the fetal head may also occur several weeks before true labor, commonly called lightening. In the majority of vaginal births, the fetal head is the "presenting part," or the body part that proceeds first in passage through the pelvic canal. Breech presentations, where the fetal pelvis or leg(s) become the presenting part, may also be delivered vaginally if they meet specific obstetrical criteria but will not be discussed in this chapter.

Once the fetal head is engaged, the fetus undergoes a series of movements and position changes called the cardinal movements of labor. These movements allow the relatively large fetal head (and body) to fit through the relatively narrow maternal pelvis by changing their orientation and position as they progress through the birth canal. The purpose of these movements is to present continuously the narrowest possible diameter of a given body part through each section of the pelvis. To facilitate its passage, the fetal head undergoes temporary "molding," a process where the head is elongated and the skull bones may overlap to decrease total head circumference by up to 2.5 centimeters. Occasionally, women may experience cephalopelvic disproportion, where the fetal head does not successfully negotiate through the maternal pelvis and labor is stalled. This can be the result of a disproportionately large fetal head, small maternal pelvis, or failure of uterine contractions and/or fetal maneuvers to allow successful progression of the fetal head through the pelvic canal.

The second stage of labor begins with full dilation of the cervix to 10 centimeters. By this time contractions are usually as frequent as every two to three minutes, lasting approximately sixty seconds. The head is said to be "crowning" when it is resting on the pelvic floor muscles, distending the vulva, and visible at the vaginal opening. By this time the mother will feel an impulse to bear down (push) with each contraction. Delivery can be considered imminent, but this phase of labor may last from twenty minutes to two hours. Gradually, the head, shoulders, body, and legs are delivered, and slow controlled expulsion is preferable in order to protect the maternal perineum (the muscular area between the vagina and the anus) and prevent injury to the fetal brachial nerve plexus (which could cause weakness or paralysis of the baby's arms). After delivery, the neonate's airway is suctioned, umbilical cord clamped, and eyedrops applied. This is when sequential Apgar scores are performed. Episiotomies (an incision through the pelvic floor musculature extending the vaginal opening either downward toward the anus or partially sideways toward the buttocks) are frequently performed in order to prevent spontaneous rupture of the maternal perineum during delivery of the head, and consistently used in the case of forceps or breech deliveries. While commonly practiced, episiotomies remain somewhat controversial due to the potential for subsequent laceration and various associated postpartum difficulties.

The third stage of labor includes inspection of the maternal perineum, vagina, and cervix for lacerations and bruising, implementation of any necessary repairs, and delivery and inspection of the placenta. The final stage of labor encompasses the hour immediately following delivery, when the mother must be closely monitored for degree of postpartum bleeding.

Cesarean Section

Cesarean deliveries are performed for a number of reasons, the most common being failure to progress in labor. They are also performed in the case of specific maternal medical conditions or illnesses, fetal distress or abnormalities, and placental abnormalities. Previously having undergone a "classical" cesarean, where the incision runs vertically along the body of the uterus, necessitates repeat cesarean delivery because of the risk of scar rupture during pregnancy and labor. Choice of particular type of cesarean delivery is based on varied maternal and fetal conditions or circumstances, such as *placenta previa* (low-lying placenta), position of the fetus in utero, and the degree of urgency of delivery. The two fundamental types of cesarean are based on location and type of uterine incision.

The classical cesarean is considered a faster procedure and simpler to perform, and may be used for urgent deliveries. It is associated with increased risk of blood loss, potential for subsequent adhesions and intestinal obstruction, and scar rupture during the next pregnancy, so is somewhat less commonly used. In this type of cesarean, an incision is made through the skin and subcutaneous tissue (under the skin) from beneath the umbilicus (belly button) to above the pubic bone, exposing the fascia (connective tissue) between the layers of abdominal muscles. This fascia and any abdominal fat are cut and the abdominal muscles pulled to either side to reveal the peritoneum (a membrane surrounding the pelvic cavity) covering the uterus. The peritoneum is cut along the same length as the abdominal incision, exposing the uterus. A small vertical incision is made through the anterior (front) uterine wall in the upper segment of the uterus, and extended downward with blunt-edged scissors. Small blood vessels are clamped or cauterized (burned at the ends to close off the vessel) throughout each layer of the incision in order to prevent excessive bleeding.

If the fetus is in a head-down position, it is delivered feet first through this incision. The placenta is then delivered and the uterus repaired. Some surgeons lift the uterus out of the pelvic cavity, resting it on the (sterile-draped) abdomen, in order to inspect, wipe out, repair, and massage it (which stimulates uterine contraction and involution, minimizing risk of subsequent hemorrhage). Tubal ligation may be easily performed in this position. The uterine incision is stitched with one or two layers of absorbable sutures. If exteriorized, the uterus is then returned to the pelvic cavity and the sequential layers of the abdominal incision are also repaired.

The most common type of C-section uses a "low transverse" incision through both the abdominal wall and the uterus. This involves a horizontal (transverse) incision through the abdominal wall several centimeters above the pubic bone (symphysis pubis), cutting through the same layers as described above, pulling apart the abdominal muscles to expose the lower portion of the uterus. A vertical abdominal incision may also be used with a transverse uterine incision, but transverse (horizontal) abdominal incisions are often preferable because they are associated with decreased risk of subsequent wound opening (called wound dehiscence) and/or hernia at the incision site. After cutting through the peritoneum, the bladder must be retracted in order to reach the desired lower segment of the uterus; the bladder is normally superimposed on and loosely connected to the lower uterus. A special bladder retractor holds the bladder away from the uterus, allowing access. A small (2 centimeters) horizontal incision is made through the lower anterior uterine wall, and then enlarged laterally (sideways) with blunt scissors or fingers into a crescent shape. The ends of this horizontal incision angle upward in order to avoid uterine blood vessels. The baby is usually delivered headfirst from this incision, sometimes requiring forceps or upward pressure through the vagina if the head is tightly wedged in the pelvic canal (as with cephalopelvic disproportion). Subsequent care of the baby and inspection and repair of the uterus and abdominal wall are the same as with the classical cesarean.

The Pelvic Floor

The term *pelvic floor* refers to the muscles that line the bottom of the pelvis, from front to back and side to side. The perineum is one segment of these muscles. The pelvic floor has three separate muscle layers from deep to superficial, and while each has specific functions they all work synergistically and as one unit to support the abdominal and pelvic organs, maintain proper anatomic position of pelvic organs in relationship to one another, maintain urinary and fecal continence, maintain contents of uterus during increases in abdominal pressure, and facilitate erection of the clitoris.

Pregnancy and vaginal birth can cause stretching and weakening of the pelvic floor muscles, as well as of supporting ligaments, leading to "stress" urinary incontinence. Normally, increases in abdominal pressure, as occur with coughing, laughing, or straining to lift, cause an involuntary compression of the bladder neck

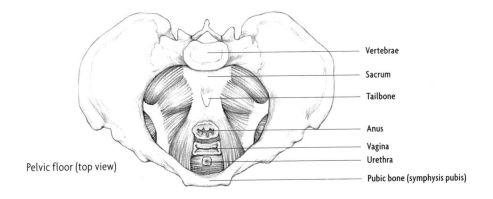

Pelvic floor (top view)

Vertebrae

Sacrum

Tailbone

Anus

Vagina

Urethra

Pubic bone (symphysis pubis)

against the symphysis pubis (pubic bone), preventing loss of urine by reinforcing closure of the urethra and the internal urinary sphincter. When pelvic floor muscles are stretched, pelvic organs, including the bladder neck, may be less well supported and descend from their ideal anatomic position. The involuntary mechanism preventing urine loss with abdominal pressure no longer occurs, and increases in abdominal pressure instead cause leakage of urine as abdominal pressure begets bladder pressure which exceeds urethral closure pressure, causing urine loss. There are other types of urinary incontinence, but stress incontinence is the type most commonly associated with pregnancy and childbirth.

Happily, much pregnancy-related and postpartum incontinence is transitory and resolves within a few months of delivery. However, many women need to actively rehabilitate these muscles in order to regain continence, and some will need to seek medical attention if the symptom persists despite their efforts. The Kegel exercise is the common name for pelvic floor exercises, which were originally developed in the 1940s by Dr. Arnold Kegel. It is said that four to six weeks of regular pelvic floor exercise may restore urinary continence by strengthening the pelvic floor muscles and muscles around the urethra, but as with any other muscular work, maintenance exercise is also required to maintain the benefits.

How to Do Pelvic Floor Exercises

The most challenging aspect of performing pelvic floor exercises is ensuring that you are contracting the right muscles. Many people make the mistake of clenching their buttocks, contracting their abdominal or inner-thigh muscles, or bearing down as if having a bowel movement rather than actual contraction of the pelvic floor musculature. With correct isolation of the pelvic floor muscles, all these peripheral muscles stay relaxed. Once you have learned to identify and isolate these specific muscles, the exercises are merely a systematic sequence of their contraction and relaxation. Tangentially, strong abdominal musculature probably contributes indirectly to urinary continence by supporting the position of pelvic contents anteriorly (in the front), but the abdominals should be relaxed during the actual performance of pelvic floor exercises.

The predominant swatch of pelvic musculature runs from front to back (pelvic bone to coccyx), so when pelvic floor muscles are contracting, the side walls of the vagina close inward, the perineum (that region of skin between the vagina and anus) pulls upward toward the body, and the flow of urine (and stool) is stopped. You can practice identification of these muscles while urinating by stopping the stream of urine; alternately, you can place one to two fingers in your vagina, squeeze as if to stop the flow of urine, and see if you feel pressure being exerted on the sides of your fingers and upward from the bottom of the vagina. Feeling the perineum move in toward the body is a little more subtle, but this is another method to verify muscle contraction. Some people feel the contraction more posteriorly, and find it easier to visualize holding back gas or stool rather than urine; in either case it is the same musculature, and contraction of the vagina produces contraction of the anus and vice versa. Again, all the peripheral muscles should be relaxed.

Once you are confident of having identified your pelvic floor muscles, you can begin daily exercises. Pelvic floor exercises can be done either seated or supine (lying flat on back). Standing places a burden on the muscles by virtue of gravity, so the muscles are not fully at rest and the exercises may be less effective and more difficult to perform. It is also more difficult to isolate pelvic muscles when you are standing.

Pelvic floor exercises include a series of short and longer contractions with at least an equal period of rest between each. There is no absolute consensus on how long to hold the contractions, but short contractions are commonly two to five seconds and longer contractions ten or more seconds. Shorter contractions tend to strengthen the types of muscle cells that use oxygen for energy and which contract involuntarily (these are the muscle cells involved in orgasm); longer contractions strengthen and help increase the muscle cells more responsible for the bulk and tone of the pelvic floor. Recommendations for the number of contractions to be performed daily vary from as little as 30 to as many as 200. A reasonable compromise might be 50 to 100 total contractions per day, which is best split into two to three shorter sessions since the muscles fatigue rapidly.

Sit in a comfortable chair with your feet flat on the floor or lie on your back with your knees straight or bent. Do a series of 10 to 15 two- to five-second contractions, resting to the same count between each. Repeat the process with the same number of ten-second (or more) contractions. Ideally, repeat this process for a total of three times per day. The sequence takes very little time, is invisible to observers, and can be performed anywhere. Longer pelvic floor contractions, as performed during *mula bandha* (see page 226), are also beneficial, but should not entirely replace the formal practice of pelvic floor exercises if being performed in an attempt to improve continence.

Once symptoms of urinary incontinence resolve, the benefits can be maintained with a once-daily practice of approximately thirty contractions; this should be done indefinitely. In addition to performing daily pelvic floor exercises, most women, even those without significant incontinence, can benefit from using pelvic floor contraction prophylactically. For instance, if you anticipate a sneeze or cough, contract and hold your pelvic floor muscles through the event. Done intentionally at first, this rapidly becomes a habit and effectively prevents episodic urine loss. Or, if you have an urgent desire to go to the bathroom and none is available, or have difficulty with frequent feelings of urinary urgency, stop and squeeze the pelvic floor muscles for as long as you can. This contraction sends a message back to the spinal cord that causes reflex inhibition of the bladder contractions initially causing the sense of urgency. The urge to void will pass and can be successfully inhibited in this way repeatedly until you are ready to void.

Incontinence can be a deeply frustrating problem, and one it might feel easier to ignore. Feelings of embarrassment about this symptom may precipitate needless withdrawal from intimate and social activities. Don't hesitate to consult with a health care professional if you suffer with frequent or severe urine loss, or if postpartum incontinence does not respond to one or two months of pelvic floor exercises. There are many effective treatment options ranging from medications to devices to surgery, and postpartum incontinence is a very treatable problem.

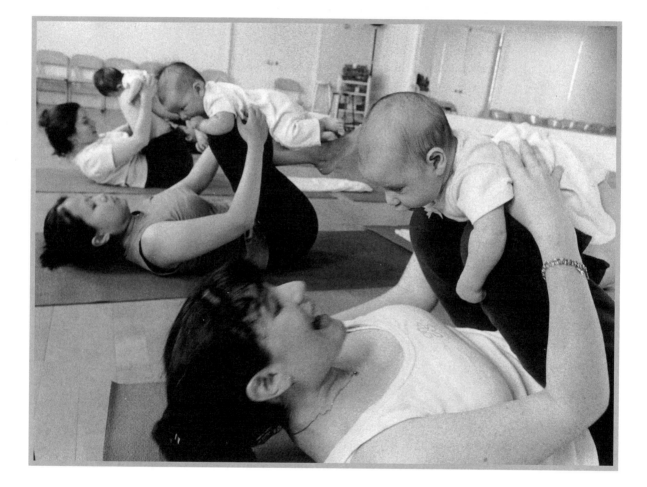

11

Postpartum Conditions

WRITTEN WITH JENNIFER STATON, M.S., N.P., R.N.,
AND ANDREW D. PERRON, M.D.

This is the most technical chapter in the book, and it's intended to serve as a resource in which you can look up specific medical issues that concern you and understand them in the context of yoga. The issues dealt with range from minor occurrences such as hair loss to much more serious problems such as diabetes. We've included this information because we believe that a good understanding of medical conditions of all types is essential to effective postpartum recovery as well as an informed and balanced yoga practice.

We must stress one thing: whatever condition you face, please make sure your health care provider gives you the green light to begin yoga, and if you suspect something is amiss, consult him or her immediately. Remember, pregnancy and childbirth exact a tremendous toll on your body and are likely to trigger hidden medical issues of some kind (usually minor, happily). For example, some of the normal physiological changes that occur in pregnancy include loosening of ligaments (caused by an increase in the hormones progesterone and relaxin), increased resting heart and respiratory rate, and an increase in blood volume and red blood cells by up to 50 percent. During your postpartum recovery such changes do resolve, but some of the conditions discussed below may be unmasked or exacerbated by them, or by other, similar factors.

We have included yoga *asanas* that might be helpful for the related condition, many of which derive from B. K. S. Iyengar's *Light on Yoga*. It is important to note that while Mr. Iyengar is unquestionably a world authority on yoga, he is not a medical doctor. He has, however, had decades of success treating people through *asana* practice.

Ankle Swelling and Pain

Ligaments are loosened during pregnancy and the ankle joints are especially vulnerable. Increased fluid and blood volume may also cause swelling, especially in the lower leg. Collapsed arches, weakened inner thighs, and pain in your knees and lower back all contribute to ankle pain and injury. Wearing an ankle brace can give some support for a weakened ankle; however, a brace will function effectively as a reminder to work carefully and should only be used on a temporary basis. There is no substitute for strengthening the muscles around the joint for lasting joint stability. Exercise helps to increase circulation, which decreases swelling. Always lift inner anklebones away from each other, especially in all the standing poses, and do ankle circles (slowly) in both directions, twelve times each day. The point and flex exercise and all *asanas* listed in the collapsed arches section are indicated. Rest, ice, compression, and elevation (Legs Up the Wall) will also help ankle swelling and pain. (See also Collapsed Arches, page 238.)

Breast Complaints

Cracked nipples: Use a lanolin-based lotion or oil on the nipple, and try nursing for less time each session. Try different nursing positions and make sure your baby has latched onto as much of each areola as possible.

Spurting nipples: When your milk lets down and your nipples begin to spray milk, press on them.

Mastitis: A bacterial infection of the milk ducts in the breast, usually caused by bacteria from the baby's mouth, characterized by an area of warmth, pain, and redness on one breast. This requires treatment with antibiotics, but you may continue to breast-feed. Emptying of the affected breast facilitates healing.

Insufficient milk supply: This can happen for several reasons. Exhaustion, poor nutrition, and dehydration are some possible culprits. Inconsistent nursing can also be a factor: if this is the case, pumping will help. Do the cesarean class (chapter 7) focusing on the *asanas* that open your chest, which are thought to increase circulation and help lactation.

Carpal Tunnel Syndrome

An inflammation of the median nerve where it passes under the ligament band that runs across the inner wrist, caused during pregnancy by excess fluid in the body. (This condition is also caused by repetitive motions such as typing.) Symptoms of carpal tunnel include wrist and hand pain and numbness, mostly along the thumb and first two fingers. This is often more bothersome at night, when muscles relax and the hands assume a flexed resting position. It can occur while you are pregnant or some months after, gradually disappearing as the hormonal shifts and edema (swelling) subside. You should not lift, flex, or strain your wrists if there is any pain. Do not do poses that require you to bear weight on wrists if you are experiencing active symptoms. When working with weight on your arms, you can fold a washcloth into quarters or roll your mat and place it under the palm of the hand, leaving the knuckles on the ground to minimize the flexion of the wrist. Plank Pose or Plank with knees on the floor will help strengthen arms and wrists but should be avoided if actively symptomatic. Commercial wrist splints can be helpful in supporting the wrists in proper anatomic position, minimizing persistent re-injury.

Collapsed Arches

Your feet can widen during pregnancy. This can occur due to ligamentous laxity (loosening of ligaments) and a change in weight distribution. In pregnancy the weight tends to shift to the outside of your legs and feet; this can weaken your inner thighs and flatten your arches. When doing standing poses, imagine an **X** on the bottom of your foot, big toe to outer heel and pinkie toe mound to inner heel, with even pressure on all four points. Separate and lift anklebones and the apex of your arch. The importance of attending to the collapsed arch also extends beyond the immediate foot area, however; it is important to build your whole posture from the bottom up. A favorite saying of one of our teachers is "what you do with your feet is what you do in the rest of the body." All standing poses are beneficial, most notably Mountain Pose, Forward Bend, Awkward Pose, Triangle Pose, Warrior II, Wide-Leg Forward Bend, and Flank Pose. A basic foot strengthener is to simply point and flex, paying special attention to articulating through the ball and toes of the foot. Others include ankle circles and spreading the toes in all standing postures.

Diabetes

Gestational diabetes occurs in up to 12 percent of pregnancies, most often in women predisposed to the condition. Family history of diabetes and current personal obesity, especially abdominal obesity, both increase risk. Because testing is performed routinely in the third trimester of pregnancy, you will no doubt be aware if you have or had this condition. Gestational diabetes usually resolves soon after delivery, but the individual remains at increased risk for developing overt Type 2 diabetes at some later point. Gestational diabetes is physiologically equivalent to adult onset or Type 2 diabetes, a condition caused primarily by the body's resistance to the effects of insulin and, to a lesser degree, by inadequate insulin production. Insulin is a hormone produced by the pancreas that allows your body to carry blood sugar into cells to nourish and stimulate energy production. Glucose is the primary fuel within the body. When insulin is either deficient or not being adequately used by the body, glucose levels rise in the blood, unable to get into the cells. This effectively causes starvation within the cells as they are not receiving nourishment despite the available unused blood sugar. The individual may unintentionally lose weight, feel increased hunger and thirst, note frequent profuse urination as the excess blood sugar pulls body fluid into the bladder like a sponge, and may notice blurred vision or a fruity odor to the breath if the blood sugar becomes excessive. Any of these symptoms should be reported to your health care provider, and the last two symptoms should be considered urgent. Regular (daily) exercise and a controlled-calorie diet are both critical in the treatment of gestational and Type 2 diabetes, and maintaining a normal weight may actually prevent it. Suggested *asanas* to practice are Head to Knee Pose, Sage Pose, Lying-Down Twist, Half Wheel Pose, Locust, Boat Pose, Forward Bend, and Resting Pose.

Diastasis Rectus

Diastasis is when a section of connective tissue between the two vertical swatches of abdominal musculature (rectus abdominii) weakens, leaving a small gap along the midline of the abdomen. This is generally considered benign but may increase the risk of abdominal (ventral) hernia. Knead your hand across your lower abdomen, pulling the muscle tissue toward the midline while you are doing any abdominal work, and tighten your abdomen by pulling gently in and up. Beware of hyperextending your rib cage in poses such as Triangle, Warrior II, and Downward Facing Dog. Focus on the cesarean Class 4 (chapter 7), which emphasizes pulling together the midline. Transition from Class 4 to Class 1—0–3 months—for a minimum of four weeks before attempting the 3–6-months class. Back bending can prevent diastasis from healing.

Episiotomy

The stitches are usually healed by the third week. Kegel exercises are safe while the incision is still healing.

Forearm Pain

This can be caused by the strain of pushing a stroller or even just by carrying your baby. Check your carrying form—it is best to carry your baby close to your own center. While practicing yoga, take care not to hyperextend the elbow. If you feel pain slightly bend the elbow. It is necessary to strengthen the biceps and triceps and the muscles of the wrists. *Asanas* indicated are Plank with knees bent, Triangle Pose, Cobra, Downward Facing Dog, and Baby Om's Sphinx Variation.

Hair Loss

Hair loss occurs after you stop nursing due to hormonal changes. Don't worry—it will grow back.

Hemorrhoids

Hemorrhoids are prolapsed anal veins caused by excessive internal pressure and pushing. They feel like little grapes around your anus, and may be painful or itchy. Sitz baths (sit in a small amount of lukewarm water), an ice compress, witch hazel, and Kegels can all help. Small amounts of blood on the toilet tissue after a bowel movement is expected with hemorrhoids, but excessive bleeding indicates a need to consult your provider. Recommended yoga poses for this are Lying-Down Twist, Full Bow, and Half Wheel.

Hernia

A hernia may occur during pregnancy because of an existing weakness in the abdominal wall exacerbated by the increased intra-abdominal pressure. This condition needs your doctor's attention. You should refrain from doing anything that puts pressure in the abdominal area (like Boat Pose) or stepping forward into Lunge from a Downward Facing Dog position. Start with Class 4, the cesarean section class, minus the Boat Pose and work carefully from there.

High Blood Pressure

Untreated high blood pressure can have serious consequences. See your doctor before beginning any exercise program. *Asanas* recommended are Downward Facing Dog, Child's Pose, Wide-Leg Stretch, and Legs Up the Wall with a pillow under your hips.

Hot Flashes

Hot flashes can occur due to hormonal changes (as in menopause). Don't worry, they will stop.

Incontinence

See pelvic floor description, page 230. Kegel exercises (*mula bandha*) are a recommended treatment.

Knee Pain

If not the result of injury or trauma, knee pain is commonly benign and caused by a variety of factors, including mechanical strain due to being overweight, quadriceps and/or hamstring weakness, arthritis, or local inflammation. Symptoms often are localized to the front of the knee with pain noted while ascending and descending stairs, after prolonged periods of inactivity, or with bending or squatting. You may initially treat this symptomatically with regular dosing of Tylenol, gentle stretching and strengthening exercises, ice massage, and avoidance of exacerbating movements. Pain that persists beyond two weeks should be evaluated by your health care provider. The following symptoms should be discussed with your provider: significant swelling of the knee (either in front or back), joint locking or buckling (giving way beneath you), difficulty walking or bearing weight on the affected leg, recurrent clicking, popping, or grinding sounds from the joint. Make sure when working in *asana* practice that you maintain a lift of the kneecap by engaging the muscles of the quadriceps. Poses to work on are Triangle Pose, Flank Pose, Wide-Leg Pose, Tree Pose, Forward Bend, and Mountain Pose. If you are not experiencing active symptoms, practice Warrior II and Lying-Down Twist.

Lower Back Pain

This is the most common musculoskeletal complaint of pregnant and post-partum women. Factors include weakened deep abdominal muscles, tucked or overarched pelvis, tight hips and thighs, tight hamstrings, and a generally stressed alignment. Nine months of being pregnant can exacerbate any already existing problems, as will carrying your baby. Essential to the support of the lower back are a correctly aligned pelvis and strong abdominal muscles. Boat Pose, Navel Sweeps, Awkward Pose, and Baby Om's Sphinx Variation are excellent abdominal strengtheners. If it is difficult to sit on the floor with straight legs due to lower-back tightness, sit on a pillow or work in the pose with bent knees. Seated poses such as Head to Knee Pose, Cow Pose, Star Pose, and Bound Angle Pose will open hips and help stretch the lower back. Other poses that help are Triangle and Wide-Leg Stretch for the spine lengthening and hip release they provide, and Child's Pose for relaxation of the lower back. Gentle twisting such as is done in Seated Twist or Lying-Down Twist will bring circulation and movement to the area. Resting Pose should be done with a pillow under knees or feet and calves on chair.

Pain around Cesarean Incision

Once your incision has healed, massage the area with vitamin E oil or another lotion. Massage can help transform scar tissue for up to 18 months postoperatively. Avoid excessive sun exposure to the scar for the first 12 months, as this can result in a darker, more noticeable scar. Avoid wide-leg standing poses, lunges, and back bends. (See chapter 7, the cesarean-section class.)

Plantar Fasciitis

Plantar fasciitis is a condition marked by heel pain (sometimes severe) when initially rising to walk after periods of inactivity; it is often improved by several minutes of walking. It is caused by a tightening of the Achilles tendon, which pulls on the fascia (connective tissue) in the sole of the foot (plantar). The pain you experience is due to micro-tears of the plantar fascia when you stand. Massage the calf and sole of the foot, and stretch the Achilles tendon and the bottom of the foot before standing to walk. Ice massage for the sole of the foot is effective for pain relief, and ibuprofen is important to relieve local inflammation. Ice massage can be accomplished by rubbing a piece of ice along your heel until the skin feels numb. Wear a comfortable flat shoe with gel heel pads inserted into the shoe. See your health care provider if this symptom persists, as it occasionally requires cortisone injections or surgery. Yoga *asanas* recommended for this condition are Downward Facing Dog, Bound Angle Pose, Child's Pose, and Legs Up the Wall.

Sciatica

Sciatica, an inflammation around the sciatic nerve, can cause pain to radiate from your lower back through the backs of one or both legs. The best thing to do is rest, apply ice, and take Tylenol. Work gently, with soft knee bends to protect against jamming in the lower back. Sometimes the pain is not sciatica but a tight piriformis that arises from the duck walk (common in pregnant women), among other things. The piriformis crosses the sciatic notch (which is in the pelvis) and if drawn taut can press on the nerve causing pain similar to sciatica, though not radiating down the leg. Use easy twisting of your spine to release the muscles around the sacrum. Try Cow Facing Pose to open the lower back, and stretch the piriformis muscle. Also indicated are Flank Pose, Triangle Pose, Side Tree, Forward Bend with bent knees, Sphinx Variation, Cobra, and Seated Spinal Twist with one leg straight. Resting Pose should be done with a pillow under your knees or feet and calves on a chair.

Shoulder Pain

Shoulder and neck pain can be referred pain from upper back weakness. Also, repetitive movements such as carrying and nursing can cause shoulder problems such as tendinitis of the rotator cuff or bursitis. Tight upper back and neck muscles such as upper trapezius, scalene, and levator scapulae can exacerbate shoulder pain, as well as the factors listed below in the upper back pain section. If joint pain is worsening, see your health care provider. Exercise is essential for joint health; it is important to stretch the pectoral muscles and strengthen the upper back. Recommended poses specifically for your shoulders are Supine Chest Opener, Cow Facing Arm Variation, and Half Wheel, as well as all *asanas* indicated for upper back pain.

Thrombophlebitis

Thrombophlebitis is a rare but potentially serious condition. There are two types of thrombophlebitis or blood clots of the lower leg, either those in the deep or in the superficial veins. The deep vein blood clots are the major cause for concern. Signs of phlebitis are redness, tenderness, and warmth in the calf along with edema below this area; flexing the foot may cause sharp pain in the front of the calf. This condition occurs most often following a cesarean delivery, and/or in cases of prolonged bed rest or inactivity. See your doctor immediately if you have pain, redness, and swelling in your lower leg. Class 4 (chapter 7) is recommended after healing is complete.

Thyroid Imbalance

The thyroid is a small gland in the front of your neck that establishes your metabolic rate. In some cases, pregnancy can affect your thyroid functioning. Increased thyroid function causes people to lose weight or feel shaky, anxious, hyper, depleted, and intolerant of heat; you may notice rapid hair loss, heart palpitations, or hand tremor. An underactive thyroid causes the opposite symptoms, including fatigue, sluggishness, low mood, cold intolerance, and constipation. Postpartum thyroiditis, an inflammatory condition of mild transient hyperthyroidism followed by mild transient hypothyroidism, is relatively common and may occur up to six months postpartum. If you suspect you may have thyroid problems, consult your health care provider; testing is simple and accurate. Indicated *asanas* are Downward Facing Dog, Half Wheel, Supine Chest Opener, and Resting Pose with legs on a chair, hips elevated on a pillow.

Upper Back Pain

Upper back pain is a common postpartum complaint. Factors include poor posture, tightened pectoral muscles, overstretched and weak upper back muscles, exhaustion, nursing, use of the baby carrier, dehydration, and lifting and carrying. All chest openers will help to stretch and realign upper body carriage. The middle trapezius and rhomboid muscles are often the most overstretched and weakened. Cobra, Locust, and Camel Pose, in which you pull the shoulder blades together, strengthen the upper back and open the chest. Also indicated are Downward Facing Dog, Triangle and Revolved Triangle, Sitting Twist, and Sage Pose. Class 2 was especially designed to address this problem, with each of the three standing poses emphasizing a back bend before the Forward Bend. This condition needs both stretching and strengthening to be effective. See also *asanas* for shoulder pain.

Varicose Veins

Varicose veins are common in pregnancy, and may or may not fully disappear. Lying-Down Twist, Handstand, and Resting Pose with legs up the wall are recommended.

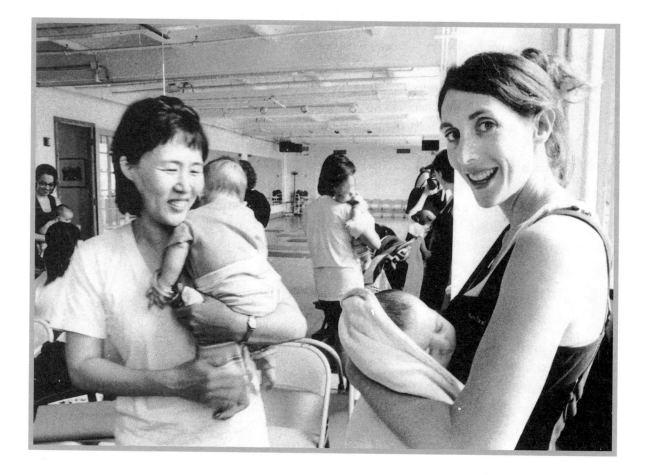

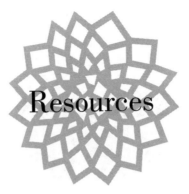

Resources

Baby Om
212-615-6935
www.babyom.com
laurastaton@yahoo.com
spmk@earthlink.com

Tools for Yoga
P.O. Box 99
Chatham, NJ 07928
888-678-9642
staff@yogapropshop.com

Hugger-Mugger
Salt Lake City, UT 84123
800-473-4888
www.huggermugger.com

Yoga Pro
P.O. Box 7612
Ann Arbor, MI 48107
800-488-8414
www.yogapro.com

Yoga Props
3055 23rd Street—J
San Francisco, CA 94110
888-856-YOGA
yogaprops@sfo.com

www.birthlight.com

www.sitaram.org

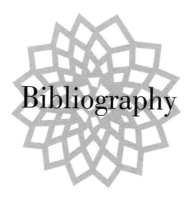

Bibliography

American Academy of Child and Adolescent Psychiatry. *Your Child: Emotional, Behavioral, and Cognitive Development from Birth through Pre-Adolescence.* New York: HarperCollins, 1998.

Brazelton, T. Berry, M.D. *Infants and Mothers: Differences in Development.* New York: Bantam Doubleday Dell, 1983.

———. *Touchpoints: The Essential Reference.* Reading, Mass.: Addison-Wesley, A Merloyd Lawrence Book, 1992.

Cunningham, F. G., et al. *William's Obstetrics,* 19th ed. East Norwalk, Conn.: Appleton & Lange, 1993.

DeCherney, A. H., and M. L. Pernoll. *Current Obstetric and Gynecologic Diagnosis and Treatment,* 8th ed. East Norwalk, Conn.: Appleton & Lange, 1994.

Eisenberg, Arlene, Heidi E. Murkoff, and Sandee E. Hathaway. *What to Expect the First Year.* New York: Workman Publishing, 1996.

Eliot, Lise, Ph.D. *What's Going On in There?* New York: Bantam, 1999.

Farhi, Donna. *The Breathing Book.* New York: Henry Holt/Owl, 1996.

———. *Yoga: Body, Mind, and Spirit.* New York: Henry Holt, 2000.

Frank, Ruella, Ph.D. *Body of Awareness: A Somatic and Developmental Approach to Psychotherapy.* New York: Gestalt Press, 2001.

Gopnick, Alison, Ph.D., Andrew N. Meltzoff, Ph.D., and Patricia K. Khul, Ph.D. *The Scientist in the Crib*. New York: William Morrow, 1999.

Hacker, N. F., and J. G. Moore. *Essentials of Obstetrics and Gynecology*, 3d ed. Philadelphia, Pa.: W. B. Saunders Company, 1998.

Iyengar, B. S. K. *Light on Yoga*. New York: Schocken Books, 1979.

Iyengar, Geeta S. *Yoga: A Gem for Women*. Spokane, Wash.: Timeless Books, 1990.

Karlowicz, K. A. *Urologic Nursing, Principles and Practice*. Philadelphia, Pa.: W. B. Saunders Company, 1995.

Lasater, Judith. *Relax and Renew: Restful Yoga for Stressful Times*. Berkeley, Calif.: Rodmell Press, 1995.

Leach, Penelope. *Your Baby and Child: From Birth to Age Five*. New York: Alfred A. Knopf/Dorling Kindersley, 1997.

Leboyer, Fredrick. *Loving Hands: The Traditional Indian Art of Baby Massage*. New York: Alfred A. Knopf, 1976.

Marieb, E. N. *Human Anatomy and Physiology*, 2d ed. Redwood City, Calif.: The Benjamin/Cummings Publishing Company, 1992.

Mehta, Shyam, and Mira Silva. *Yoga: The Iyengar Way*. New York: Alfred A. Knopf/Borzoi, 1995.

Noble, Elizabeth. *Essential Exercises for the Child-Bearing Year*. Boston: Houghton-Mifflin, 1982.

O'Brien, Paddy. *Yoga for Women*. New York: HarperCollins/Thorsons, 1991.

Ramaswami, Srivatsa. *Yoga for the Three Stages of Life*. Rochester, Vt.: Inner Traditions International, 2000.

Stern, Daniel N., M.D. *Diary of a Baby*. New York: Basic Books/Perseus, 1998.

Walker, Peter. *The Book of Baby Massage: For a Happier Healthier Child*. London: Kensington Books, 1988.

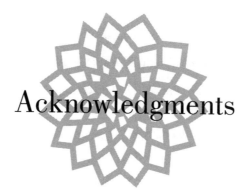

Acknowledgments

We are deeply grateful to the artists who worked with us making this book a reality. Josh Titus, whose charm, talent, and photographs shone for the duration of the project, Anja Hitzenberger for her dynamic movement-charged images, Hugo Martin for his playful and lovely drawings, Jennifer Staton for her keen skepticism and fierce skill, Johanna Simpson for her compassion and insight, Andrew Perron for his doctor's acumen, and Ruella Frank for her deep commitment to physical and mental health.

Many thanks to our families, Diana and Robert Perron, Patricia Hodge, Sharon Engberg, and Rita Stanko for their ongoing support. Heartfelt thanks to Fuensanta Gutierrez for introducing us to her methods and to her teachers Diana de La Rosa and Nora Trejo, from whom we have learned so much. We would also like to thank our friends whose insight helped guide us many times over, notably Mari Lazar, who always came to our rescue when we needed it, Andrew Raible, who had all the contacts, and Rob Bresserer, Hilary Buchanan, Marina Budhos, Rachel Lynch-John, Linda Lynn, Carole and Lisa Margolin, Susan Ordahl, Lee Polychron and Howard Coale, Karen Schwartz, Howie Seligmann, and Deborah Wolfe.

We wish to thank Billie Fitzgerald for selling our idea, Anja Jankowsky for her Baby Om Web site, and Maria Robledo and Holton for generously donating their loft for our photo shoots. Also many thanks to Jeanne-Marie Derrick for consulting with us and sharing her expertise. Thank you to Debra Goldstein, our agent at Creative Culture, for being a tireless advocate, our editor

Deborah Brody, who gave us the latitude and guidance to realize the book we envisioned, and Ellen Greenfield, who pulled it all together.

We are greatly indebted to our teachers, present and past, who have inspired and nurtured us: Genny Kapular, Jeanne-Marie Derrick, Carol Foster, Robin Janis, Alison West, and Sharon Gannon, among others.

We also wish to thank our students, who have shared their babies' first year with us, and especially those who have modeled and written for this book: Alex King and Maya, Karen Wallace and Ella, Katrina Cunningham and Teagan, Andrea Taetle and Katie, Debra Fraser and Molly, Barrie Raffel and Shane, Bibi Calderaro and Nina, Emily Schmalholtz and Justin, Alyssa Gilbert and Rosie and Sam, Grace Offitt and Madeleine, Sarah Kapocias and Maddie, Mari Lazar and Zoe, Tina Fehlandt and Sam, Michelle So and Kaitlin, Jennifer Gerakaris and Nikki, Sarah Verdone and Louisa, Camilla Essner and Mindy Zelen and Jenna, Pam Tanowitz and Jemma, Rebbeca Todd and Duncan, Jenny Siahaan and Batara, Margot Hasker and Isabella, Liza Napier and Aiden, Elizabeth Kaiden and Simon and Eva, Gallit Hasak and Eli, Rachel Sarah and Mae, Amy Sirot and Ben, Naomi Goldberg and Noah, Nitza Wilon and Sam, Susan Ordahl and Trygve and Elsa, Natasha Grigorov and Uma, Sarah Burnes and Gideon, Katrin Schnabel and Sebastian, and Yunah Hong and Ejun.

Grateful thanks to Miles Parker whose birth informed the creation of this book in two distinct ways: first, the ongoing wealth of information he generated at a time when we most needed it and second, for his dazzling and photogenic grin.

Last, we want to thank our husbands—Michael Kaniecki, whose enthusiasm and support made the long hours possible, and Neil Parker, whose unflagging involvement, skill, and good taste helped us create a better book.

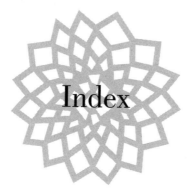

Index

Page numbers in italics indicate main entries for exercises. The italic *f* denotes an illustration.

Full Wheel (*Urdhva Dhanurasana*), 121,
   159–61, 160f
fussy babies, 211

Gate Pose (*Parighasana*), 121, *150–51, 150f*
gestational diabetes, 238–39
glucose, 238
grabbing, 124
grasping, 27, 124

hair loss, 80, 235, 240
Half Wheel Pose (*Setu Bandasana*), 33, 69–70,
   70f, 81, *112–13, 112f, 155–57, 156f,* 161,
   180–82, 181f
   baby engagement in, 71–72, 113–15, *157,*
     182
   for diabetes, 239
   for postpartum conditions, 244, 245
Half Wheel Spine Rolls, 213
hamstrings
   variation for warming: Standing Forward
     Bend, 53, 199
   variation to stretch: Side Tree, 189
hand-eye coordination, 82, 195
hands, weight-bearing, 18
Hands on the Floor, *28, 28f*
Handstand (*Adho Mukha Vrksasana*), 47,
   146–48, 147f
Handstand preparation, *145f*
head (baby), supporting, 82
head and neck control, 26, 37, 38
Head to Knee Pose (*Janu Sirsasana*), 33,
   62–63, 62f, 104–5, 104f
   for diabetes, 239
   for postpartum conditions, 242
healing, 7, 11
health care provider, 235, 239, 241, 243, 244,
   245
heel pain, 243
hemorrhoids, 19, 240
hernia, 230, 239, 240
high blood pressure, 241
holding baby, 25
hopelessness, 217, 218, 220
hot flashes, 241
hyperthyroidism/hypothyroidism, 244–45

ibuprofen, 243
identity, sense of (baby), 82
incision (cesarean), 174, 229, 230
   pain around, 175, 242
incontinence, 241
   see also urinary incontinence
inhalation, 15, 17, 34, 125
insulin, 238
interpersonal connections, 83
intestinal distress, 211
Iyengar, B. K. S., 236
Iyengar, Geeta, 164

joint rotation exercises, 38
joint squeeze
   ankle, *27f*
   arm, *27f*
joints, 35

Kegel, Arnold, 231
Kegel exercise (*mula bandha*), 7, 17, 34, 40, 57,
   80–81, 85, 126, 175, 188, 190, 226, 231,
   240, 241
   with episiotomy, 239
kicking (baby), 82
Knee Crawling, *153, 153f*
knee pain, 241–42
Knuckle Rub, *27, 27f*

labor, 173, 176, 226, 227–28
   failure to progress, 173, 229
   stages of, 227–28
leg extensions, 88
leg rotations, 89
leg(s)
   variation: Locust Pose, 106
   variation to strengthen: Half Wheel Pose,
     157
Legs Up the Wall (*Savasana*), *206–7, 207f,*
   236
   for postpartum conditions, 241, 243
Leopard Swing, *58, 58f,* 212
Lewis, Victoria, 3
ligaments, 35, 230
   loosening of, 235, 236, 238
Light on Yoga (Iyengar), 236